What They Are Saying About This Book

"a 'gem'!"

"*Never Smoke Again* is a very complete and easy to read resource. It will be extremely useful to persons seeking to stop smoking and to their family members and loved ones who want to help them kick the habit. It will make great reading material for any health care clinic to assist people in knowing what resources are available to help stop smoking efforts and how to put those resources into practical use. It is definitely a 'gem'!"

Debra Romberger, MD
Professor of Internal Medicine,
Section of Pulmonary and Critical Care,
University of Nebraska Medical Center

"the best investment you can make"

"*Never Smoke Again* is the perfect gift for a loved one or close friend who would like to stop smoking but can't. Dr. Grant Cooper explains why smoking is such a dangerous habit, why quitting is so beneficial to the smoker and his contacts, and the various techniques that can improve the odds of quitting. He does this in a sympathetic and non-preachy style. This may be the best investment you can make."

Steven A. Schroeder, MD
Distinguished Professor of Health and Health Care,
Department of Medicine Director,
Smoking Cessation Leadership Center—
University of California, San Francisco

W9-AXZ-035

NEVER SMOKE AGAIN

The Top 10 Ways to Stop Smoking Now & Forever

GRANT COOPER, MD

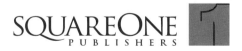

SQUAREONE
PUBLISHERS

The information and advice in this book are based on the training, personal experiences, and research of the author. Its contents are current and accurate; however, the information presented is not intended to replace professional medical advice. The author and the publisher urge you to consult with your physician or other qualified health-care provider prior to using any smoking-cessation method. Because a risk is sometimes involved, the author and publisher cannot be responsible for any adverse effects or consequences resulting from the use of any of the quitting methods described in this book.

COVER DESIGNER: Jeannie Tudor
IN-HOUSE EDITORS: Joanne Abrams and Marie Caratozzolo
TYPESETTER: Gary A. Rosenberg

Square One Publishers
115 Herricks Road
Garden City Park, NY 11040
(516) 535-2010 • (877) 900-BOOK
www.squareonepublishers.com

Library of Congress Cataloging-in-Publication Data

Cooper, Grant, M.D.
    Never smoke again : the top 10 ways to stop smoking now and forever /
Grant Cooper.
        p. cm.
    Includes index.
    ISBN 978-0-7570-0235-9 (pbk.)
    1. Smoking cessation—Popular works. 2. Nicotine addiction—Treatment—
Popular works. I. Title.

RC567.C68   2007
616.86'506—dc22
                                                                2007008208

Printed in the United States of America

10   9   8   7   6   5   4   3   2   1

Contents

I dedicate this book to my Uncle Alan,
who quit smoking more than twenty years ago.
Since that time, he has lived more, seen more,
and done more than he had imagined possible.
He continues to mentor and inspire me.

Acknowledgments

There are many people who made this book possible. First and foremost, I would like to thank my wife, Ana. Ana provides the foundation for all that I do. Her thoughtful comments and revisions for this book were indispensable.

Thank you, too, to Rudy Shur, the head of Square One Publishers. He has been a joy to work with and I admire his commitment to excellence. I am also very grateful to Joanne Abrams and Marie Caratozzolo of Square One Publishers for their outstanding work in editing this manuscript.

Thank you to my parents, who continue to be my base of unwavering support. Their counsel guides me through all that I do.

Thank you to my parents-in-law, who encourage and challenge me to always think, write, and debate the "real things."

Thank you to Jason, Sharon, Aaron, Viktor, Robin, John, Emma, and Allison for inspiring me, each in their own way.

Introduction

Y ou've done it! By deciding to read this book, you have taken a signifi- cant step toward breaking your addiction to cigarettes, and are on the way to a tobacco-free life. Maybe you've tried quitting before, only to return to cigarettes after days, weeks, or even months of being smoking-free. But be assured that you *can* stop smoking. In fact, according to the American Lung Association, well over 45 million Americans have already quit. How did they do it? They found the method that worked for them and they stuck with it. Often, it wasn't the first method they had tried. In fact, most smok- ers attempt to quit several times before they are successful—before they find the technique that works for them. This book was designed to guide you in finding the quitting method that's right for you so that you will never smoke again.

Will quitting be easy? No. Early in my life, I learned just how addictive cigarettes can be. My uncle was at death's door over twenty years ago. Not yet forty-five years of age, he had heart problems and ultimately had to undergo triple bypass surgery. Still, he smoked. My aunt couldn't under- stand why he was slowly killing himself, but no matter how he tried, he couldn't kick the habit. Finally, his doctor told him, "Alan, if you don't quit smoking, you'll be dead in seven years." Something clicked, and he never picked up a cigarette again.

The good news is that it's not necessary to face a life-threatening con- dition to quit smoking. Once you understand how cigarettes snare you, and what they do not only to your health but also to the health of your loved ones, it becomes clear that you *have* to quit. That's why Part One of *Never Smoke Again* begins by taking a long, hard look at cigarettes, why we smoke them, and how they keep us coming back for more, even when we want

1

desperately to toss them away. It then discusses the many health consequences of tobacco—consequences that go far beyond respiratory illness and lung cancer. Finally, Part One prepares you for your Quit Date by helping you access your core values and cement your resolve. By the time you finish the last page, you'll be ready to stop for good!

Part Two is about making that all-important choice of anti-smoking techniques. In each of ten chapters, you'll learn about one of the top ten methods of quitting, including cold turkey; tapering off; nicotine patches, gum, lozenges, nasal spray, and inhaler; Zyban; Chantix; and hypnosis. What exactly is each method? How does it work? How do you use it? What are its risks and drawbacks? And, perhaps most important, does it work? In each case, you'll find answers to these questions, along with proven tips to help you succeed. Special Pros and Cons sections highlight the important features of each technique, making it easier to pick the tool or tools most suited to your needs.

As you read about the various quitting techniques now available, one of the most important things you'll learn is that these techniques do not necessarily have to be used singly, but can often be combined. Quitting experts, for instance, often recommend pairing a nicotine replacement therapy like the patch with a prescription aid such as Zyban. This can greatly increase your chance of success. And, of course, hypnosis—a drug-free therapy—can be combined with any of the other techniques to further strengthen your resolve and keep your motivation high. Remember this as you design your own stop-smoking program, because a smart blend of tools may be just what you need. But also be aware that these tools should *never* be combined without the help of your doctor, as an unwise mix can cause problems. In fact, before beginning any anti-smoking program—even one that relies on over-the-counter aids—it is a good idea to consult with your physician. Besides making the quitting process safer, a doctor's expert guidance can also make it far more effective.

Throughout this book, I emphasize that knowledge is power, and that support is key to success. That's why *Never Smoke Again* ends with a list of Resources, including organizations that can supply further information; in-person, online, and phone support; quitting guidelines; and much more. A world of assistance is just a mouse click or phone call away. Don't overlook all the valuable help that has been made available to you.

Although *Never Smoke Again* provides the information you need to choose the quitting method that's right for you, it's important to understand that no method or combination of methods, no matter how effective, can quit for you. You have to approach the quitting process with firm resolve, and you have to be ready to work toward your goal. But make no mistake about it: You *can* stop smoking. You have within you the strength necessary to kick the habit. *Never Smoke Again* will show you how to access that power, team it up with a proven quitting technique, and begin a new, healthy, cigarette-free life.

PART ONE

What You Should Know

How Did You Get Here?

Can you remember why you started smoking? Was it to be cool? Was it to fit in with your friends who smoked? Did you believe it was part of your "coming of age"? Did you think it was sexy? Did it signify your independence? How did you get hooked? And why is it so difficult to quit?

This chapter begins with a look at the advertising industry's past and present roles in glamorizing smoking. It explains their many tactics, both obvious and subtle, that successfully lure people into getting hooked. The chapter concludes with an informative discussion of addiction—one of the major reasons it is so difficult to quit smoking.

THE ADVERTISING INDUSTRY

Stop and consider where your image of smoking came from. When did inhaling thousands of toxic, cancer-causing fumes become the image of cool? For most people, the answer to that question is simple. It came from advertising. Your image of cigarettes (one you may not even be aware of) has been carefully cultivated by highly paid, skilled marketing executives who are employed by multi-billion dollar tobacco corporations. These marketing moguls sure know what they're doing. Their ads don't paint honest pictures of cigarettes—what they contain and the harm that they cause. Have you ever seen an ad from a tobacco company which mentions that when you inhale cigarette smoke, you are taking in some of the same chemicals that are used to kill rodents?

During the 1950s and 1960s, cigarette ads, whether in the form of television commercials, print ads in newspapers and magazines, or larger-than-life advertisements on outdoor billboards, were always alluring, always appealing, and usually targeting a specific audience. There was the macho "Marlboro Man," a rugged cowboy with a cigarette dangling from his mouth—an image that personified manliness. In the 1960s, the introduction of Virginia Slims brand cigarettes and its "You've Come a Long Way, Baby" campaign targeted the growing population of women smokers by appealing to their sense of independence. Advertisers had a field day with catchy cigarette slogans and popular jingles like "Winston Tastes Good Like a Cigarette Should," "L&M. Just What the Doctor Ordered," and "Us Tareyton Smokers Would Rather Fight Than Switch."

There was also "Joe Camel," a cigarette-smoking cartoon camel. Supposedly, this image was created to attract younger smokers (mostly between ages eighteen and twenty-four) to choose the Camel brand. The amiable cartoon character also appealed to very young children. In 1991, an article published in the *Journal of American Medical Association* revealed that children who were six years old were able to recognize Joe Camel more than 90 percent of the time—about as often as they were able to identify the Mickey Mouse logo used on the Disney television channel. The article also concluded that it was the intention of the campaign to directly market to children. In 1997, under increasing criticism and pressure from anti-smoking groups, the Federal Trade Commission, and the U.S. Congress, R.J. Reynolds (the makers of Camel cigarettes) voluntarily ended the use of Joe Camel in its ads.

In 1970, the U.S. Congress passed a law that banned the advertising of cigarettes and other tobacco products on radio and television. Print ads in magazines were still permitted; however, all advertisements, as well as product packages, were required to display a health warning from the Surgeon General. Not being able to advertise on TV may have been a setback for tobacco companies, but it was a minor one. They continued to promote their products in indirect, more subtle ways.

What were some of the ways tobacco companies began to indirectly advertise? For starters, they found great success in creating "ads" of their products by embedding them in movies. Lois Lane did not smoke in the

Who Is the Real Marlboro Man?

Among the many actor/models who have portrayed the Marlboro Man in print and television ads, two have died from lung cancer. Wayne McLaren was one of them. Before his death at age fifty-one, McLaren started an anti-smoking campaign, which included a powerful television commercial that juxtaposed images of him as the Marlboro cowboy with those of him in his hospital bed.

Superman comic book series, but she chain-smoked Marlboros all through the movie *Superman II.* That same movie showed the Marlboro brand approximately forty times, including a scene in which Superman threw the evil villain Zod into a Marlboro truck. Phillip Morris reportedly paid $42,000 for that placement—a mere pittance considering the number of people it reached.

Phillip Morris wasn't alone. Between 1988 and 1997, more than 85 percent of each year's top twenty-five films included tobacco use, often targeting specific brands. In the Walt Disney movie *Who Framed Roger Rabbit?* the main character smokes Lucky Strikes. The father in *Honey I Shrunk the Kids* tries to quit his addiction to Camel cigarettes, which are in the camera's clear view. *Ghostbusters II* includes packs of both Marlboros and Kools.

The power of this form of subliminal advertising is strong. According to Robert Kovoloff of Associated Film Promotions, "Seeing a product, even for a second, in a realistically dramatic setting in which the viewer is already emotionally involved leaves an invaluable impression." And young people under age twenty, who make up about 40 percent of moviegoers, are especially susceptible to being influenced by what they see on the big screen. To serve as an example, after Reese's Pieces were spotlighted in the movie *ET: The Extra-Terrestrial,* sales for the candy skyrocketed. The reality is that these cigarette placements in movies send a more powerful message than print ads. They certainly make more of an impression on young people, who want to look like, dress like, and smoke like their favorite celebrities.

In 1998, a legal agreement in forty-six states ensured that tobacco companies could no longer legally pay for product placement in movies. And yet, due to loopholes in the agreement, tobacco "impressions" continue to make their way to movie audiences.

Other indirect methods of advertising used by the tobacco industry include sponsorships of live (often televised) sports events, direct-mail campaigns, special sales promos, and catchy point-of-sale displays. Another advertising tactic is the use of tobacco brand names on non-tobacco products, such as the Marlboro Classics clothing line—a wide range of shirts, jackets, and accessories that include the logos and/or ads associated with the Marlboro brand.

The bottom line is this: Tobacco companies invest significant capital to make you think of positive images—sexiness, beauty, independence, intelligence, wealth, popularity—every time you see a cigarette. They're betting that these associations will make you more likely to put your money down on their product. Guess what? They're right. The more you associate tobacco products with positive attributes, the more likely you are to buy cigarettes. Furthermore, they're betting that if they can hook you when you're young, you'll become a lifelong customer.

Don't let them get away with it. Don't allow yourself to be manipulated. In order to change both your conscious and subconscious perceptions of smoking, it's important that you perceive reality. Whenever you see cigarettes, try to see them for what they *really* are—cancer sticks, instruments of heart disease, toxic-fume delivery systems. When you see a beautiful woman putting a cigarette to her lips, don't imagine that she looks cool or sexy as the smoke billows from her lungs and circulates lazily into the air. Remove that mental image from your mind and picture what is really happening. Instead of a cigarette, imagine that the woman is wrapping her lips around the exhaust pipe of a car. Envision the arsenic, carbon monoxide, acetone, benzene, and thousands of other toxic, cancer-causing chemicals filling her mouth, then coursing their way to her lungs. Imagine how they are damaging her healthy cells and compromising her well-being. When she exhales, envision the pollutant-filled smoke poisoning the air. *That's* the reality. *That's* the perception you must maintain.

Don't allow the tobacco companies to paint a false picture in your mind. When you see what is really happening, the picture is nowhere near as attractive. Paint reality—it is your friend and will help you break your emotional attachment and physical addiction to cigarettes.

NICOTINE ADDICTION

You really want to quit. You've already tried to stop a number of times, but failed. Why is it so difficult? More important, why would you continue to engage in an action that you *know* compromises your health and is likely killing you? An action that also wrinkles your skin, stains your teeth, gives you bad breath, and costs a lot of money? The truth is, you probably would not continue the action unless you were addicted to it.

Smoking is more than just a bad habit. Unlike biting nails or cracking knuckles, smoking is also an addiction, both physically and psychologically. Any addiction implies dependence, and in the case of cigarettes, the physical dependence is on nicotine. When nicotine is inhaled, it enters the bloodstream through the lungs. In the brain, nicotine increases the level of dopamine—a chemical that is responsible for feelings of pleasure and well-being. Essentially, nicotine is like candy for the brain; every puff of deadly cigarette smoke rewards the brain's pleasure center. Because these pleasurable effects of nicotine wear off quickly, people continue to smoke to maintain those enjoyable effects. And therein lies the dependence.

Interestingly, smokers have to develop a *tolerance* to nicotine. Think about the first time you puffed on a cigarette. Remember how you coughed as your body tried to reject the smoke, and how you suddenly felt nauseous and dizzy? Remember that as you continued to smoke, you were able to puff away without feeling sick? This is because your body began to build a tolerance to the nicotine, which, as mentioned in the paragraph above, eventually began to stimulate your brain's pleasure center, resulting in addiction.

When the "smoking-pleasure-smoking" cycle is broken, the result is *withdrawal*, another characteristic of addiction. Cutting off that source of pleasure causes the body to rebel. What follows is a list of commonly reported symptoms of smoking withdrawal. Be aware that most people experience some, but rarely all of them.

Anxiety	Depression	Hunger
Concentration difficulties	Dizziness	Insomnia
Constipation	Dry mouth	Irritability
Cough	Fatigue	Postnasal drip
Cravings to smoke	Headache	Sore throat

It is important to understand why you may be experiencing these symptoms. Basically, you and your body are adjusting to life without a steady flow of nicotine. If you are feeling tired and fatigued, be aware that your body is no longer experiencing the stimulant effects of nicotine. You may also find that you are hungry all the time. Perhaps this is because once you stopped smoking, your sense of taste began to improve and food started tasting better. You may have also used cigarettes as an appetite suppressant—lighting up to curb the desire to eat. Now, without cigarettes, your desire for food has increased. Instead of popping food into your mouth whenever you crave a cigarette, try to distract yourself by taking a walk or calling a friend. If you find yourself constantly coughing or experiencing dry mouth, postnasal drip, or headaches, don't be alarmed. These are signs that your body is ridding itself of the many toxins that have accumulated from smoking over the years. Finally, you can be sure that you will experience cravings for cigarettes. They may be strong, last as long as five minutes, and occur frequently. The good news is that over time, these cravings will lessen in intensity and occur less often. You must learn to get through them. Take some deep breaths, sip water or juice, go for a short walk, or find another way to distract yourself. Constantly reminding yourself of the reasons you have given up smoking will help you cope with all of these withdrawal symptoms.

An Addiction So Strong

For some people, nicotine is more addictive than cocaine or even heroin. Dr. Sigmund Freud discovered this the hard way. Early in his life, Freud, who was a cigarette smoker, became addicted to cocaine, which he had used to self-medicate his own depression. (At the time, use of the drug was legal.) He eventually stopped using cocaine, but was never able to stop smoking—even after developing cancer in his jaw, which lead to the implantation of an artificial one.

It's no secret that the power of nicotine addiction is undeniably strong. When trying to quit, be realistic—understand that you are up against a formidable opponent. Also realize that it *can* be beaten. You have the ability to do so.

Although dealing with the side effects of withdrawal can be difficult and challenging, the good news is they are only temporary. Most symptoms begin to lessen within a period of days and may last only a week or two. If, however, you find that they persist for prolonged periods or you are concerned about a physical reaction you are having, be sure to contact your health care provider. Also keep in mind that, unlike withdrawal from drugs and other chemicals, nicotine withdrawal is not dangerous. It may be unpleasant and uncomfortable, but not dangerous. And it will get better. It will get easier.

As you break free from your addiction to nicotine, your brain and body will stop rebelling, stop punishing you. The withdrawal symptoms will subside as your body adjusts to its new "smokeless" existence. The clouds will begin to lift and you will realize that you *can* make it to the other side—to the world of nonsmokers. Once there, it's important not to fool yourself into believing that you can go back to smoking "just once in a while." You can never have "just one cigarette." One will undoubtedly lead to two, which will lead to three, which will lead you back to square one. Once you quit, it's important to stay that way.

Now, let's get back to the original question posed in this chapter: How did you get here? You were swept there by the alluring pull of advertisers and their appealing images of smoking, coupled with the stronghold of addiction. Fortunately, you have the power to quit (everyone does), and the information in this book will help you succeed. The next chapter presents another very important aspect of smoking—health consequences.

Health Consequences

The last chapter helped you understand why you started smoking, how you became addicted, and why it can be so difficult to quit. In your heart, you know that it's time to free yourself of your dependence on cigarettes. That's why you are reading this book. You can't ignore the fire in your gut that is telling you to break the addiction. This chapter, which focuses on the health consequences of smoking, will help add fuel to that fire. And you're going to need that fuel to help internalize your desire for change—a critical part of the foundation of your success.

MORE THAN A BAD HABIT

In 1964, U.S. Surgeon General Luther Terry submitted his landmark report on smoking and health. The report implicated cigarette smoking as a cause of lung and larynx (voice box) cancer in men and a suspected cause of lung cancer in women. Smoking was also cited as a cause of chronic bronchitis in both sexes. This report marked the first official significant step in raising public awareness of the health ramifications of tobacco smoking. In the decades preceding the report, smoking was actually touted as being good for you—and tobacco companies, with their deep pockets, paid advertisers handsomely to aggressively spread the word. Doctors were often spotlighted in ads, puffing away on cigarettes or holding up packs, while claiming that they helped you relax, or aided digestion, or made you feel refreshed.

That first Surgeon General's report kick-started what would become a long, but significant road in the development of anti-smoking campaigns, research coalitions, and information clearinghouses. On behalf of public health, the first warning label to appear on cigarette packs—"CAUTION:

CIGARETTE SMOKING MAY BE HARMFUL TO YOUR HEALTH"—was a direct result of this milestone report.

After 1964, mounting medical research and scientific investigations began to uncover an ever-growing number of diseases and conditions associated with smoking. Soon, cigarettes were no longer linked solely to lung cancer and cancer of the larynx. They were implicated in cardiovascular disease, compromised reproduction, and cancers of the bladder, esophagus, mouth, and throat.

In 2004, forty years after that first report, Surgeon General Richard H. Carmona released *The Health Consequences of Smoking,* a comprehensive work that was prepared by nearly two dozen top doctors, scientists, and public health experts over the course of three years. The report concluded that smoking has a negative effect on just about every organ of the body. It conclusively linked smoking to such conditions and diseases as cataracts, pneumonia, acute myeloid leukemia, periodontitis, and cancers of the stomach, pancreas, cervix, and kidney. According to Dr. Carmona, "The toxins from cigarette smoke go everywhere the blood flows." The report concluded that "Smoking remains the leading cause of preventable death and has negative health impacts on people at all stages of life. It harms unborn babies, infants, children, adolescents, adults, and seniors."

The adverse health consequences from smoking cigarettes are implicated in over 400,000 deaths each year in the United States. That's an amazing one in every five deaths! Later in this chapter, you will be taking a closer look at how cigarette smoke compromises health. After all, if you are currently a smoker, this information is directly related to you. But first, it's important to understand the ingredients contained in cigarette smoke.

According to the Centers for Disease Control and Prevention, cigarette smoking is the single most preventable cause of premature death in the United States.

What's in That Cigarette Smoke?

To better understand why cigarette smoking has such a strong negative impact on health, let's take a look at what is actually in tobacco smoke.

Boasting an impressive array of "villains," cigarette smoke contains over 4,000 chemicals, including more than 60 known carcinogenic (cancer-causing) substances. The content and concentration of these chemicals vary, depending on a variety of factors, including the brand or type of cigarette. The following list contains just a fraction of the harmful contents found in tobacco smoke:

❑ **Acetone.** Highly reactive chemical often used as a cleaning agent and paint stripper.

❑ **Arsenic.** Poisonous metallic element used in insecticides and weed killers.

❑ **Benzene.** Flammable petroleum-derived liquid used in cleaning products and gasoline.

❑ **Butadiene.** Flammable hydrocarbon, derived from petroleum and used in the manufacture of synthetic rubber products.

❑ **Carbon monoxide.** Colorless, odorless, toxic gas contained in vehicle exhaust.

❑ **Cyanide.** Poisonous chemical compound used in gas chambers for executions in the United States.

❑ **DDT.** Colorless toxic insecticide.

❑ **Dieldrin.** Highly hazardous chemical used in insecticides.

❑ **Formaldehyde.** Gaseous compound used in the manufacture of dyes, fertilizers, and embalming fluids.

❑ **Lead.** Metallic element found in paint, solder, and certain types of glass.

❑ **Napthalene.** Carcinogenic hydrocarbon derived from coal tar or petroleum. Commonly used as a solvent and to make mothballs.

❑ **Styrene.** Oily compound used to make plastics such as polystyrene (Styrofoam).

❑ **Vinyl chloride.** Flammable gas used in the production of plastics.

Cigarette smoke also contains tar—the sticky brown substance made up of the particles and harmful byproducts of tobacco. It is tar that stains the teeth, fingernails, and lungs. Another major ingredient is nicotine, which is contained in the moisture of the tobacco leaf. When the cigarette is lit, the nicotine evaporates and attaches itself to minute droplets in the tobacco smoke. Nicotine is not cancer-causing, but it is toxic. It is also highly addictive, which is the main reason people continue to smoke.

Finally, don't kid yourself into thinking that low-tar or low-nicotine cigarettes offer health benefits over regular, full-flavored varieties. According to the 2004 Surgeon General's report, "There is no safe cigarette, whether it is called 'light,' 'ultra-light,' or any other name. The science is clear: the only way to avoid the hazards of smoking is to quit completely or to never start smoking." (See "Are Any Cigarettes Safe?" on page 17.)

Now be honest with yourself. If you walked into a room and the air was filled with pesticides and other poisonous chemicals, would you close the door behind you and willingly take a deep breath? Of course not. Well, that's exactly what you are doing every time you puff on a cigarette.

WIDESPREAD HEALTH DESTRUCTION

As you know, when you inhale cigarette smoke, thousands of toxic ingredients—many of which are known carcinogens—course through your body. As explained in the 2004 Surgeon General's report, these toxins go everywhere your blood flows, causing widespread destruction. They affect the proper functioning of internal organs and compromise the efficiency of the body's immune system.

Cigarette smoke contains carbon monoxide (CO)—often in high levels. Because this toxic gas binds to the hemoglobin in red blood cells, it reduces the blood's ability to carry oxygen. A heavy smoker's oxygen-carrying capability of the blood may be reduced by as much as 15 percent.

The carcinogenic agents in tobacco smoke are capable of damaging the genes that control cell growth. As a result, the cells can begin to grow either abnormally or too quickly, resulting in the formation of tumors. Healthy bodies produce antioxidants, which help repair damaged cells. Smokers have been found to have lower levels of antioxidants than nonsmokers.

Smoking is a known cause of *oxidative stress*—an oxidation process that has a negative effect on cell function and is associated with high levels of chronic inflammation. This disturbance promotes a variety of diseases, including atherosclerosis and chronic lung disease. It is also believed to be a contributor to the development of cancer and cardiovascular disease, as well as an integral part of the aging process.

As discussed in the last chapter, nicotine—the addictive component of cigarettes—makes its way to the pleasure center of the brain within seconds of that first drag. It also travels throughout the entire body and is even found in the breast milk of nursing mothers who smoke. It is also found in the semen of male smokers. (More about this in the following section.)

Are Any Cigarettes Safe?

Misled by the implied promise of reduced toxicity, many smokers believe that smoking cigarettes that are low-yield (those with reduced levels of tar or nicotine), all-natural, hand-rolled, and/or menthol are safer than smoking regular varieties. Don't believe it. *All* cigarette smoke, no matter what type of cigarette it comes from, is dangerous to the body.

Compared to *regular* or *full-flavored* cigarettes, which yield more than 15 milligrams of tar, cigarettes that are marketed as *light* (6 to 15 milligrams) or *ultra-light* (1 to 6 milligrams) are not any safer. Studies have shown that the risk for developing lung cancer isn't any lower with low-yield cigarettes, which also have little (if any) effect on lowering the risk of other respiratory illnesses or heart disease. People who switch to these brands often wind up smoking more cigarettes. They also tend to take deeper drags and smoke more of each cigarette.

All-natural cigarettes, which come in full-flavored, light, and ultra-light varieties, are advertised as having no chemicals or additives. They are also rolled with 100-percent cotton filters. Although this type of cigarette may sound like a safe alternative to consumers, there is no evidence of its safety. Like the smoke from all other cigarettes, the smoke from all-natural brands contains numerous toxins and carcinogens—including carbon monoxide and tar—that come from the tobacco itself.

The same goes for hand-rolled cigarettes. Although they may, in fact, be less expensive than manufactured cigarettes, they still produce the same poisonous smoke. Furthermore, people who smoke hand-rolled cigarettes are at greater risk for developing cancers of the mouth, throat, larynx, and esophagus.

Menthol cigarettes, which account for about 25 percent of the cigarettes sold in the United States, are not safer than other brands. In fact, studies indicate that they may actually pose greater bodily harm. When inhaled, the mentholated smoke has a cooling effect on the throat. It also represses the cough reflex and masks the dryness many smokers feel in their throats. Because of this, people who smoke menthol cigarettes tend to inhale deeply and hold the smoke in longer.

In an effort to make their smoking habit safer, some people try to reduce the number of cigarettes they smoke each day. Although this may sound like a good solution, most smokers find it difficult to follow. Furthermore, research has shown that even smoking as few as one to four cigarettes a day can result in serious heath problems, including heart disease.

It really doesn't matter which brand or type of cigarette you smoke. Nor does it matter the number of cigarettes you use each day. The bottom line is clear. All cigarette smoke is harmful to your health.

Now, let's take a closer look at some of the specific illnesses and health conditions that are linked to smoking.

Smoking-Related Illnesses and Conditions

When most people think of health issues caused by smoking, lung cancer, emphysema, and bronchitis usually come to mind. While respiratory ill-nesses are certainly linked to smoking, they are just one area of impact. As you will see, smoking is detrimental to nearly all aspects of health.

Although you might think lung cancer is the number-one killer of smokers, you'd be wrong. Coronary artery disease (also called coronary heart disease) and stroke—the main types of cardiovascular disease caused by smoking—are the country's first and third leading causes of death. Smoking has a number of negative effects on the cardiovascular system. For starters, it lowers the body's HDL ("good") cholesterol. It also wears down the elasticity of the aorta, which, in turn, increases the risk of developing blood clots. This can obstruct blood flow and result in a heart attack or stroke. Toxins in cigarette smoke cause inflammation of artery walls and contribute to atherosclerosis—hardening of the arteries. Smoking also stimulates the sympathetic nervous system, which puts undo stress on the cardiovascular system—particularly the heart and blood vessels.

Cancer is the country's second leading cause of death, with lung can-cer the most prevalent type. Cigarette smoking is responsible for nearly 85 percent of lung cancer cases in the United States. It also accounts for over 60 percent of cancers of the mouth, pharynx, larynx, and esophagus. (Those who smoke pipes or cigars, and/or chew smokeless tobacco are at great risk for cancers of the mouth and pharynx, as well.) Cigarette smokers also experience a higher incidence of acute myeloid leukemia, and cancers of the bladder, kidney, pancreas, and stomach. Women who smoke have an increased risk of developing cervical cancer.

Cigarette smoking is the most significant risk factor for chronic bron-chitis and emphysema, which are considered chronic obstructive pul-monary diseases (COPDs). These slow-progressing lung disorders cause the airways to become irritated and swollen, eventually resulting in a grad-ual loss of lung function. COPDs are the country's fourth leading cause of death, of which 90 percent are attributed to smoking.

Tobacco's negative effect on periodontal health is another area that is well documented. According to a recent study, smokers are more likely to have periodontitis (advanced gum disease) than those who have never smoked. The study found that people who smoked less than ten cigarettes a day were about three times more likely to develop periodontitis than non-smokers. Those who smoked more than a pack and a half a day had about six times the risk. Furthermore, because smoking compromises the immune system and reduces the delivery of oxygen and nutrients throughout the body, smokers often do not respond well to treatments for oral problems.

People who smoke are more likely than nonsmokers to develop cataracts; they are also at higher risk for macular degeneration. Smoking restricts blood vessels, making it difficult for oxygen and nutrients to reach the skin. Because of this, smokers tend to have a pale, unhealthy pallor. They also develop more and deeper wrinkles as they age.

Because smoking impairs the formation of new bone, women who smoke are at an exceptionally high risk for developing osteoporosis. They are also more susceptible to spinal injuries. Postmenopausal women who smoke have lower bone density than women who have never smoked. They are also at greater risk for hip fractures.

Rapid heartbeat, shortness of breath, and fatigue are common feelings experienced by many smokers when physically exerting themselves. And the term "physically exerting" can cover a wide range of activities—from running the bases during a softball game, to carrying a heavy bag of groceries to the car, to simply walking up a flight of stairs. While such reduced athletic capabilities may not seem serious, they are significant signs of smoking's undeniable effects.

Smokers also tend to incur more medical costs than nonsmokers. Due to compromised immune systems and delayed wound healing, they have lower post-surgical survival rates. They are also more likely to experience complications following surgery, such as infections and respiratory problems like pneumonia.

> In the United States, the current annual cost of health-care expenditures caused by smoking is approximately $96 billion. The expenses caused solely by secondhand smoke exposure have reached nearly $5 billion.

A person's risk of contracting any of these smoking-related diseases and conditions increases with the length of time he or she continues to smoke, and with the number of cigarettes smoked. There is, however, good news. As you will see later in this chapter, when a person quits smoking, most of these risks steadily decrease as the body gradually begins to repair the damage caused by cigarettes.

Smoking and Reproductive Health

Cigarette smoking can have extensive negative effects on all phases of reproduction. It can impede the fertility of both men and women, result in high-risk pregnancy with increased probability of complications, and compromise the health of the child.

Studies have shown that women who smoke may find it more difficult to become pregnant, with their chances of success reduced as much as 40 percent per menstrual cycle. Even low levels of smoking—including secondary smoke—can have an effect on fertility. Male smokers often have lowered sperm counts and increased numbers of damaged or malformed sperm. Also, when by-products of nicotine are present in the semen of smokers, sperm motility is reduced.

Although it has long been known that smoking during pregnancy can be harmful to both mothers and their babies, many pregnant women continue to smoke. These women are twice as likely to experience complications such as *placentia previa* (a condition in which the placenta grows too close to the opening of the cervix) or *placental abruption* (a condition in which the placenta separates prematurely from the uterine wall). Both disorders can cause a woman to hemorrhage during her pregnancy, leading to possible premature delivery, stillbirth, or early infant death. Excessive bleeding can also lead to serious complications for the mother, such as kidney failure and labored breathing. Pregnant women who smoke are also at higher risk for the premature rupturing of membranes before labor begins—an event that can result in a preterm birth.

Nicotine constricts the blood vessels in the umbilical cord and womb, decreasing the amount of oxygen delivered to the unborn baby. Cigarette smoke also slows the blood flow in the placenta, restricting the nutrients that reach the growing fetus. As a result, babies born to women who smoked during pregnancy often have low birth weights (the more cigarettes smoked, the greater the probable birth-weight reduction). Typically, low birth-weight babies have less muscle mass and more fat than babies of nonsmokers. They are also at greater risk for contracting childhood illnesses. Low birth weight is also one of the leading causes of infant death.

Sudden Infant Death Syndrome (SIDS) is the unexplained, unexpected, sudden death of an infant during the first year of life. It is also the leading cause of death in otherwise healthy infants over one month old. Although the causes of SIDS are not completely understood, according to the 2004 and 2006 Surgeon General reports, several factors clearly increase its risk. Studies have shown that chemicals in secondhand smoke affect the brain in a way that interferes with the regulation of infants' breathing. (A detailed discussion of secondhand smoke appears below.) Studies have also found that infants who die from SIDS have higher concentrations of nicotine in their lungs and higher levels of cotine (a biological marker for secondhand smoke exposure) than infants who die from other causes. The reports conclude that smoking during pregnancy is a cause of SIDS, and infants who are exposed to secondhand smoke are also at risk. Infants who are exposed to secondhand smoke *and* whose mothers smoked during pregnancy are at especially high risk. In the words of the Surgeon General, "Babies whose mothers smoke during and after birth are three to four times more likely to die from SIDS."

The detrimental effects of cigarette smoking are extensive, reaching all phases of reproduction. And secondhand smoke plays an insidious role in the compromised health of infants and children, as well. The following section takes a closer look at secondhand smoke and its long list of health implications.

SECONDHAND SMOKE

Secondhand smoke, also known as *passive smoke, involuntary smoke,* and *environmental tobacco smoke (ETS),* is a mixture of *sidestream smoke*—which is emitted from the burning end of a cigarette, pipe, or cigar—and the smoke that is exhaled by smokers. Earlier, you saw the effects of this noxious mixture on infants and children. Unfortunately, the damage caused by this smoke doesn't end there.

Secondhand smoke is a toxic blend of the same chemicals and carcinogenic compounds found in *mainstream smoke*—the smoke that is inhaled directly from a cigarette. (See "What's in That Cigarette Smoke?" on page 14.) So serious is secondhand smoke that Surgeon General C. Everett Koop brought it to the public's attention in the 1986 report *The Health Consequences of Involuntary Smoking.* In it, he exposed secondhand smoke's link to lung cancer and cardiac disease, as well as its impact on the health of children.

By 1993, the Environmental Protection Agency (EPA) had concluded that secondary smoke posed risks similar to those of mainstream smoke,

Kiss Those Nutrients Good-Bye!

It's no secret that cigarette smoke has an enormous impact on health, increasing the risk of such diseases and conditions as cancer, coronary artery disease, respiratory and circulatory problems, periodontitis, and osteoporosis. What you may *not* realize is that smoking also robs the body of a number of important vitamins and minerals—the more you smoke, the more you lose. It also affects the body's ability to absorb these essential nutrients.

Vitamin C is the primary nutrient affected by cigarette smoke. It helps boost the immune system, is needed for maintaining healthy bones and teeth, and is essential for healing wounds. Vitamin C is also necessary to form collagen, a protein that is required to make blood vessels, skin, scar tissue, and ligaments. As one of the body's many antioxidants, vitamin C helps block some of the damage caused by free radicals.

To counteract the cell damage caused by cigarette smoke, your body needs increased levels of vitamin C—which is actually stolen by that same smoke! The best solution, of course, is simply to quit smoking. Otherwise, it is important to take a daily vitamin C supplement—up to 2,000 milligrams. It is also advisable to eat vitamin C-rich foods, such as citrus fruits and juices, blueberries, cantaloupe, cranberries, mango, papaya, pineapple, raspberries, strawberries, and watermelon. Other excellent sources of vitamin C include bell peppers, Brussels sprouts, cabbage, cauliflower, broccoli, leafy greens, sweet potatoes, tomatoes, white potatoes, and winter squash.

Please keep in mind that while taking nutritional supplements can help protect your body against the damage caused by smoking, no amount can offer full protection. There is only one real solution: Kiss those cigarettes good-bye.

and actually classified it as a Group A carcinogen. This designation means there is sufficient evidence that the substance causes cancer in humans. (Asbestos and radon are among other Group A carcinogens.) The EPA report confirmed the earlier Surgeon General's report that exposure to secondhand smoke can cause lung cancer in adults who do not smoke. It also confirmed that children, whose bodies are still in a stage of physical development, are at heightened risk for certain illnesses when regularly exposed to high levels of secondhand smoke. Such exposure can cause asthma in otherwise healthy children who have not previously exhibited symptoms of the disorder. It can also trigger asthma attacks, increase their frequency, and intensify the symptoms. Infants and children who are regularly exposed to secondhand smoke experience an increased incidence of bronchitis, pneumonia, and other lower respiratory tract infections. They are also at higher risk for developing middle ear infections. And, as seen earlier, secondhand smoke plays a role in Sudden Infant Death Syndrome.

In 2006, Surgeon General Richard Carmona submitted another extensive report substantiating earlier claims regarding the impact of secondary smoking on health. The report implicated secondhand smoke in 3,000 deaths from lung cancer, 46,000 from coronary artery disease, and 430 from SIDS in the previous year. It also offered scientific evidence indicating that "there is no risk-free level of exposure to secondhand smoke." The report concluded that even short exposure to secondhand smoke can have immediate adverse health effects, particularly on the cardiovascular and respiratory systems.

Fortunately, due to growing public awareness, the country has made great strides in reducing the exposure of nonsmokers to secondhand smoke—with bans on smoking in public places continuing to grow. Unfortunately, secondhand smoke still remains a public health hazard. Many people are still exposed to it at home, in the workplace, and in places such as restaurants and bars. It is important to understand that half-hearted attempts to protect nonsmokers—separating them from smokers in the same airspace, having ventilated areas for smokers in the workplace, cleaning the air in buildings—simply won't work. Only smoke-free environments are effective. Period.

IT'S NEVER TOO LATE TO QUIT

Considering tobacco's ravaging effects on your body, you might think it is too late to quit. But you would be wrong. When you stop smoking, your body will begin to experience beneficial health changes almost immediately. And these changes will continue for years. The sooner you quit, the sooner you will reduce your chance of getting cancer or another smoking-related illness.

Imagine that you have just taken the final puff of your last cigarette. Your body will react with the following changes:

❏ **After 20 minutes:** Your heart rate and blood pressure will drop and return to normal.

❏ **After 8 hours:** The nicotine levels in your blood will be reduced by half, as will the levels of carbon monoxide. The oxygen level in your blood will increase to a normal level.

❏ **After 24 hours:** The carbon monoxide in your blood will be gone. Your lungs will begin clearing out the mucus and debris that has been building up since you started smoking.

❏ **After 48 hours:** All of the nicotine in your body will be gone. Your sense of taste and smell will begin to improve, and any damaged nerve endings will start to regrow.

❏ **After 72 hours:** Your bronchial tubes will begin to relax and breathing will become easier. You will also notice an increase in your energy level.

❏ **After 2 weeks:** Your circulation will begin to improve and your lung function will start to increase.

❏ **After 1 month:** You will begin to experience improved breathing as your lung function continues to strengthen. You will also start to notice a decrease in coughing, congestion, shortness of breath, and general level of fatigue.

❏ **After 1 year:** Your risk of developing coronary artery disease will be half that of a person who smokes.

❏ **After 2 years:** At this point, your risk of relapsing back to smoking drops sharply.

❏ **After 5 years:** Your risk of having a stroke will be the same as that of a person who has never smoked.

❏ **After 10 years:** Your risk of lung cancer will drop to half that of a person who smokes. You will also have a decreased risk of getting ulcers, and developing cancer of the bladder, cervix, esophagus, mouth, pancreas, and throat.

❏ **After 15 years:** Your risk of coronary artery disease will be the same as that of a person who has never smoked.

When you say good-bye to cigarettes, you will also be saying good-bye to stained teeth and fingernails, bad breath, and clothes and hair that reek of smoke. Quitting cigarettes also prevents the premature wrinkling of your skin. Your food will taste better, your sense of smell will return to normal, and you will be able to attack everyday activities with renewed energy. Best of all, you will *feel* better.

Some people are concerned with the possibility of gaining weight after giving up smoking. It is true that a number of smokers gain an average of six to eight pounds after they have quit smoking. Compared to all of the health risks you'll be leaving behind, this weight gain is a minor concern. View it as a challenge that can be eliminated with proper diet and exercise. Remember, if you have the strength and willpower to quit smoking, you also have the ability to deal with a few extra pounds. And don't forget, your improved lung function and overall increase in energy are likely to make exercising an easy, enjoyable activity.

Consider the words of India's spiritual leader Mahatma Gandhi who said, "Men often become what they believe themselves to be. If I believe I cannot do something, it makes me incapable of doing it. But when I believe I can, then I acquire the ability to do it even if I didn't have it in the beginning. . . . We must become the change we want to see."

SOME FINAL WORDS

Hopefully, this chapter has been an eye opener for you. Like most people, you may have thought lung cancer and heart disease were the only serious health problems caused by smoking. You may have also minimized the hazards of secondhand smoke. Now you know the frightening reality. The damage caused by all types of cigarette smoke is extensive, affecting nearly every part of the body.

But you also learned that once you quit smoking, the damage will begin to reverse itself, with some changes occurring within minutes of that last cigarette. It is never too late to quit. And the next chapter will help get you ready to break free of the addiction.

Getting Ready

Do you realize that you enjoy smoking because you have conditioned yourself to enjoy it? You have convinced yourself that you need cigarettes, making it hard to say good-bye to them.

Over time, you and your cigarettes have developed a pretty solid relationship, and it's more than just a physical addiction. Years of smoking have also created a psychological dependence—one that you have come to associate with feelings of pleasure. Cigarettes reward you after a long day at work, cap off the end of a good meal, and help calm you down when you're feeling anxious. You have come to think of cigarettes as your friends, and like friends, you enjoy having them around . . . when you're driving in the car or talking on the phone or taking a walk in the park. It's going to be hard to say good-bye to such close friends, and it's important for you to realize just how difficult it will be. But you *can* do it.

You can start by trying to maintain a realistic view of this so-called pleasurable friendship—and all that it is costing you. In addition to the physical damage cigarettes cause, don't forget about their seductive side, which keeps you dependent on them. You *need* cigarettes, so your life revolves around them. You *want* cigarettes, so they control you. Be honest. How often have you found yourself in a panic over whether you have enough cigarettes to make it through the day? How many times have you run out in the torrential rain or during a snowstorm just to buy a fresh pack? Do cigarettes always seem to be a "priority purchase" over everything else? Have you ever picked one of your stale cigarette butts from an ashtray and relit it because it was all that was around? Face it, these so-called friends own you! *They* are in control. They've got you by the throat and are calling all the shots. What kind of friendship is that? And let's not forget about the cost! You have to pay a lot of money to maintain this friendship—for both the cigarettes themselves and for all the damage that they cause. And I'm not referring solely to medical bills. How many times has a hot cigarette ash burned a hole in your clothing, or a piece of furniture, or the interior of your car? Some friend!

This chapter is designed to help you build a solid foundation that will support you as you prepare to break away from this formidable enemy that is only disguised as your friend. Setting this foundation is critical for increasing your odds of successfully quitting. First you will be taking an honest look at yourself to determine your core values. This is a necessary step to help you internalize your desire for change. Then you will receive helpful guidelines for setting a Quit Date, for building a support group to help bolster your efforts, and for staying on track. In your heart, you know that it is time to quit smoking. You want to. You have to. Most important, *you can!*

RECOGNIZING YOUR CORE VALUES

Let's face it. In order to successfully quit smoking, first and foremost, you must really want to quit. How can you internalize this desire for change? By first understanding—and I mean truly understanding—why you want to change. Only then, can you internalize that desire and translate it into action. Because you will be living and breathing that desire every minute of every day, the change will become inevitable. In fact, because the yearning to change comes from deep within, it won't even require conscious effort. How can you accomplish such an effective change in your behavior? By knowing yourself.

Once, the Greek words *gnothi se auton*, translated as "know thyself," hung over the entrance to the ancient Temple of Apollo at Delphi. These words have been attributed to a number of ancient philosophers, including Socrates. What does it mean to know thyself, and how can it help you quit smoking?

Lasting change needs strong, enduring willpower or desire, which requires constant energy to stay strong. If your desire is weak or superficial and doesn't come from a place of renewable energy, it will quickly burn itself out. This means that your desire to change must come from deep within yourself, where energy is fed from an inherent strength in your soul. Everyone has this strength, but not everyone finds a way to access it. "Look well into thyself," said Roman Emperor Marcus Aurelius. "There is a source of strength which will always spring up if thou wilt look there." From such a place, you cannot help but be victorious over any vice.

In order to know thyself—to harness the great power you hold within your soul—you must take the time to recognize what matters to you most. In their best-selling book *The Power of Full Engagement,* Jim Loehr and Tony Schwartz describe their approach to helping people make effective, lasting changes in their personal and professional lives. One of the first steps is to identify your core values—the essential principles that define a person's character. Integrity, compassion, honesty, fitness, and courage are just a few examples of core values. Identifying yours will help you achieve a greater sense of purpose. It will also make everyday decisions in your life easier because they will be consistent with your personal values.

Let's say, for example, that one of your core values is to live with integrity. If you took your family to a restaurant and discovered that the waiter had forgotten to charge you for one of the entrées, you wouldn't think twice about what to do. Even if the service was slow or the food was overpriced, your core value of integrity would guide your decision to alert the waiter of his error. Your decision is a no-brainer because it's the only choice consistent with integrity. Actually, it's not even a choice; it's an action that is simply a manifestation of who you are.

You might believe that being healthy is one of your core values, but your two-pack-a-day habit makes you question that belief. Don't. Because you have never taken the time to properly identify your core values, your actions may not necessarily reflect them. That's part of the problem! Now is the time for you to do so as you embark on one of the most important changes in your life.

Perhaps one of your core values is "staying healthy so you can be there for your family." Once you have honestly identified this, your decision of what to do when you pass a store that sells cigarettes is easy. Since smoking is obviously not consistent with staying healthy, you no longer have to fight the urge to run into the store and buy a pack. There is only one urge, one voice that is guided by this core value—and it is telling you to keep on walking. The weight and energy of trying to will yourself to avoid going into the store is gone. You walk past it because you have no choice. It is the only way you can be true to yourself.

So how can you determine your core values? Some people find it easy to look into their souls and make this honest assessment. Others find it more difficult. Let me share a college experience that helped me recognize some of my own principles. You might find it helpful as well.

One of my psychology professors started the class one day by asking us to think about things that were important to us. After a minute or so, we had come up with answers such as grades, dating, friends, money, and our favorite sports teams. Then she turned off the lights and asked us to close our eyes. She told us to imagine that our lives were over and we were lying in a coffin six feet under the ground. She instructed us to hold that image in our minds and think of nothing else. With our eyes closed, we sat in silence for about five minutes, all the while imagining we were dead. When the professor's voice eventually broke the silence, she asked us once again to consider what was important to us. This time, in the quiet calmness of our innermost selves, our thoughts turned to our families, friendship, honesty, integrity, and living a good life.

I found the exercise to be a soul-searching experience. If you feel that you have not adequately connected to your own inner values—the principles that guide you as a person—this might be a good exercise to try. Death will come to us all. How do you want to live? What is truly important to you? Figure that out by knowing thyself. Identify your core values, and the rest will flow easily from there.

SETTING A QUIT DATE

Once your resolve to kiss those cigarettes good-bye is firm and internalized, it's time to decide on a Quit Date—the first day of your smoke-free life. It is the day you reclaim control of your future . . . the day your body can begin to reverse the damage caused by cigarettes.

It's best to pick a date within a week or two of your decision to quit, while your resolve is still fresh and strong. If you wait any longer, you run the risk of losing your momentum. And you will need all the strength and drive you can muster. Once you've chosen the date, circle it on your calendar and tell your family and friends. You're going to need their support. It's also time to seriously begin thinking about which quitting method to use. Will you be relying solely on willpower and try to stop cold turkey? Will you be using a stop-smoking aid, such as the nicotine patch? Are you considering hypnosis as a quitting tool? Part Two, beginning on page 39, presents valuable information on these and other effective stop-smoking methods. Take the time to learn about them, including their pros and cons. It will help you decide which method (or methods) might best suit your particular needs.

During the days leading up to your Quit Date, there are a number of ways you can begin to prepare yourself. Start by making a list of all the reasons you want to quit and carry it with you at all times. Whenever you find yourself with a free moment—during a break at work, while stopped at a red light, when standing in line at the bank—take it out and read it. While your list is likely to include health-related reasons, don't forget to add the more personal ones, like living long enough to see your daughter get married or being around to enjoy your grandchildren.

As your Quit Date draws near, consider switching to a different brand of cigarettes—preferably one you don't like. If you smoke regular cigarettes, for instance, switch to menthol; or if you smoke full-flavored cigarettes, switch to ultra-lights. And no more cartons! Buy only one pack at a time. Also try to limit your smoking to certain places, such as outdoors.

Start stocking up on items that will help get you through those first few weeks of cravings. Sunflower seeds, chewing gum, lollipops, carrot and celery sticks, raisins, and hard candies are just a few popular choices. Some people find it helpful to chew on straws or swizzle sticks. Holding these items will also keeps your hands busy, replacing the urge to hold a cigarette.

Another helpful idea is to gather together some pictures of the people who mean the most to you—those who may be your inspiration for quitting cigarettes. Post the pictures on your refrigerator, on your desk at work, on the visor of your car, anywhere you will see them during the day. Also consider posting a picture that reminds you of how you do *not* want to look—someone with yellow teeth and wrinkled skin from years of smoking, or a person who is hooked up to an oxygen mask or lying in a hospital bed. Reminders such as these will keep you strong in your resolve to quit.

Make the day before your Quit Date a cleanup day. Get rid of all your ashtrays at home and work. (I recommend throwing them out!) Clean out the ashtray in your car. Throw out your empty cigarette packs. Open the windows and air out your house. It will take awhile for the smell of stale smoke to disappear from your curtains and carpeting, but it will happen eventually. For the same reason, have your clothes cleaned, including coats and jackets. (Think about how nice it's going to be to have fresh breath and hair that doesn't reek of stale cigarette smoke!)

Before your Quit Date, you might map out a way to reward yourself for reaching certain milestones once you've quit. Plan to treat yourself to something special when you've gotten through the first day, the first week, the first month of not smoking. Believe it or not, incentives such as these can help keep you focused. And *anything* that prevents you from giving in to the urge to smoke is worth trying.

Successful quitting takes planning and commitment. Preparing for your Quit Date is critical. Mentally and physically it helps you get ready to face the challenge. This means you have to be aware of the possible withdrawal symptoms that lie ahead. You must expect the cravings that will challenge your will and weaken your desire to quit. (You must also know that these symptoms are temporary.) Knowing what to expect can help you prepare to face the enemy head on.

Beginning with that first day as a nonsmoker, try to keep as active as possible. When you feel that enticing, often intense urge to reach for a cigarette, distract yourself with a brisk walk, a bike ride, or a swim. Go to the local batting cage or driving range, or toss a football around with your kids or next-door neighbor. Take a trip to the mall, the library, or the park. In other words, do *anything* that helps distract you from the urge to smoke. Be sure to drink lots of water or juice, which will also help curb the cravings. You can also take deep breaths, just as you did when inhaling a cigarette. Only during this breathing exercise, remind yourself of the reasons you have quit smoking.

Let's Talk Dollars and Cents

If you need more than the fear of a heart attack or lung cancer to throw out those cigarettes for good, maybe the incredible amount of money your habit is costing will be just the incentive you need. It's a real eye-opener!

Let's start with the cost of cigarettes themselves. While the price per pack varies in this country from state to state and from brand to brand, currently, the average cost is around $5.00. This means, if you are a two-pack-a-day smoker, you're shelling out about $10.00 a day, $70.00 a week, $280.00 a month, and $3,360.00 a year on cigarettes! That's a nice amount of cash—cash that you could put toward buying a new car, or taking a much-needed vacation, or making a sound investment.

To discover how much you personally spend on cigarettes over the course of time, visit the website of the American Cancer Society at *www.cancer.org* and type "tobacco cost calculator" into the search box. This site also provides a "cigarette calculator" that tallies up the number of cigarettes you smoke over a specific period.

But the monetary consequences of smoking go far beyond the cost of the cigarettes themselves. For obvious reasons, smokers pay more for life insurance premiums than nonsmokers (some policies cost more than double). Many homeowners' insurance policies reward nonsmokers with discounted rates, and

Be sure to avoid situations in which you typically feel the urge to smoke. Stay away from any triggers (and this can mean people) that encourage you to light up. Eventually, you will be able to face these situations with a renewed sense of strength and confidence, but it's best to avoid them during the fragile first few weeks or so of quitting. Also consider changing your daily routine—take an alternate route to work or school, go out for breakfast instead of eating home, or set aside part of your lunch hour to take a short walk.

The day you quit smoking can be likened to jumping into a pool of cold water. It will be jarring at first, but if you stick with it, your body will eventually acclimate to its surroundings. Soon you will find yourself actually enjoying the water. Relapsing can be compared to getting out of the water. Once you're out, even if it's just for one cigarette, getting back in is going to require that jarring experience again. So jump in, and give it your best effort to stay in.

---

in a growing number of states, government employees who smoke have to pay more for their health insurance benefits.

Your habit could also affect your paycheck! In most states, employers are able to discriminate against both potential and current employees who smoke. This means that in addition to implementing a "no-smoking" workplace environment, companies can refuse to hire people who smoke—and they have! A number are even subjecting their current employees to nicotine tests. Face it, smokers are at a higher risk for compromised health, costing their employers more in productivity and sick days. So more and more companies are responding with these types of anti-smoking policies.

Now think about all of the extra money you are spending at the dry cleaners to get the stale smell of cigarette smoke out of your clothing, and at the dentist to brighten your ever-yellowing teeth. Also think about how much you spend each week on breath mints. Even your house or apartment requires additional cleaning costs to get rid of the smell that has settled into curtains and carpets. (If you happen to be selling your house, be aware that a house that smells of cigarette smoke is a turnoff to potential buyers.)

So it isn't just the cost of a pack of cigarettes that's affecting your wallet. Your habit is a constant drain on many areas of your life. Of course, while this dollars-and-cents aspect is certainly something to consider, never forget smoking's most serious cost—life itself.

BUILDING A SUPPORT GROUP

Dealing with all of the physical and psychological challenges that are an inevitable part of the quit-smoking experience is not an easy task. Even with the help of the anti smoking aids presented in Part Two, you can find yourself ready to give up. That's why it is very important to have a support team in place to help keep you on track.

Depending on an individual's needs, a support team can be large or small. And everyone's needs are different. If you are like most people, you will want to rely on friends and family, particularly those you live with or see often. The first step is making them aware of your decision to quit smoking. Let them know that you need their support. Just knowing that they are aware of what you are going through will be helpful. They will be there for you, helping to keep you occupied and distracted during moments of weakness.

You might know of someone—perhaps a relative, friend, or coworker—who also wants to quit smoking. If he or she is as serious about quitting as you are, you might enlist that person as a "quitting buddy," which can be a great addition to your support team. Ex-smokers are another valuable source of both strength and comfort. Because they have walked in your shoes and know first-hand how hard it is to quit, ex-smokers tend to be compassionate and are likely to encourage your efforts with great enthusiasm. They may even offer new tips and suggestions that have worked for them.

I also recommend that you speak to your health care provider about your desire to quit. He or she may be able to offer helpful suggestions, and guide you in choosing the best stop-smoking method, whether it's cold turkey, a form of nicotine replacement therapy, or a combination of different aids. Although many of these aids are sold over-the-counter, they may not necessarily be safe for you, especially if you use more than one. This is why it is advisable to check with your doctor first, and follow his or her advice.

Becoming part of a quit-smoking program or support group will enhance your chances of quitting and staying that way. For programs in your area or on the Internet, check with your health care provider or contact organizations such as the American Lung Association and the American Cancer Society. You can also contact the North American Quitline Consortium (1-800-QUIT-NOW) for telephone counseling. Beginning on page 143, the Resources section offers a list of smoking-cessation programs and support groups.

Yes, your support team—no matter how large or small—can be a wonderful source of strength when you quit smoking. But no matter how fantastic your team is, ultimately, you are the only one who is accountable for your actions. You alone have to step up and follow through on the commitment to break away from cigarettes forever. Others can only offer their help.

FALLING OFF THE WAGON

American writer and humorist Mark Twain once said, "It's easy to quit smoking. I've done it hundreds of times." This amusing thought, unfortunately, can be echoed by lots of people who have tried to give up cigarettes. Many successful former smokers made several attempts to quit smoking before giving up cigarettes for good.

According to the National Center for Chronic Disease Prevention and Health Promotion, most relapses occur within the first three months after quitting. During the first week, when your body is still addicted to nicotine, it may be especially difficult. Withdrawal symptoms and cravings to smoke are generally the strongest during these first few days. Be prepared for this difficult time, and plan to use whatever resources you have at your disposal. If you make it through that first week without smoking, congratulations. But you're certainly not out of the woods. Although your physical addiction to nicotine may be gone, your psychological dependence is still very much alive and can be easily triggered. That's why it is so important to stay focused and to maintain your desire to remain smoke-free.

But what happens if you break down and smoke, in spite of all of your efforts? Well, you can do one of two things. You can either decide to start smoking again, or you can refocus and renew your commitment to quit. Choosing the latter is not going to be easy, but think about all the time and effort you have already invested in quitting. Try not to allow yourself to waste all that you've done. Don't give in to those cigarettes. You really don't want to become a slave to them again, do you?

As a general life lesson, everyone fails at one thing or another. What's important is to learn from those failures. Consider a businessman who is so paralyzed by the fear of losing money that he fails to act on obvious opportunities. How successful can he be? If that same person tries and fails, as long as he learns from his failure, he has a better chance of succeeding in the future. When motivational speaker Anthony Robbins was starting out, he wanted to talk in front of audiences as often as possible. By speaking over and over again, he was able to make mistakes, learn from them, and improve. Now, he is a world-renowned performer and life coach.

This same concept applies to quitting cigarettes. If you should relapse, don't view it as a complete failure. Look at it as a learning experience. Why did you fall off the wagon? What caused the relapse? What was the trigger that caused you to light up again? Make a careful, honest evaluation of what went wrong, and then try to prevent it from happening again. Perhaps you tried to quit cold turkey, but found the withdrawal symptoms too much to handle. If so, maybe you should consider using a nicotine-replacement aid to help wean you off cigarettes. If you lost control and decided to light up because you were among friends who smoke, it might be a good idea to avoid hanging around them for awhile—just until you're feeling stronger about your commitment. If this isn't possible, at least try to maintain a realistic vision of what is happening when you see them light up. As they puff away, try to envision the tobacco smoke eating away at their lungs and damaging their hearts. Is this really what you want for yourself?

If you started smoking again simply because you lost your enthusiasm for quitting, you may need to get back in touch with your core values. Spend some quiet time alone, thinking about all that is really important to you. Hopefully, this will help you regain your desire to quit with renewed spirit and vigor.

What's most important is that you don't give up on yourself (and give in to those cigarettes!) just because you've relapsed during a moment of weakness. Remember the sage words of renowned political leader Nelson Mandela: "The greatest glory in living lies not in never falling, but in rising every time we fall."

THE NEXT STEP

Now that you have come to the end of Part One, hopefully, you are feeling armed and ready to do battle against cigarettes—that formidable foe you once thought of as your friend. You have the willpower, confidence, and strong desire to make this life-saving change.

It's time now to choose a stop-smoking method. In an effort to help you make an informed decision, Part Two presents detailed information on the ten most effective techniques. Keep in mind that while the quitting aids presented on the following pages can be effective tools that support you in your effort, you can't rely on them to do all the work. Think of them only as an integral part of your support team—a team over which *you* alone are in charge.

PART TWO

The Top Ten Stop-Smoking Methods

#1

Cold Turkey

One of the best-known ways to quit smoking, and possibly the most popular, is going "cold turkey." With this method, you simply toss out your cigarettes and stop smoking. No pills. No patches. No aids of any kind.

You won't find a lot of advertisements for quitting cold turkey. After all, there is no drug to take or product to sell. There is no company to pay for television commercials or magazine ads. But for many smokers, quitting cold turkey has proven to be the best solution. Is it the best solution for you, too? Let's learn a little bit more about the cold turkey method.

WHAT IS IT?

The essence of quitting cold turkey is to pick a Quit Date and stick to it. When you wake up on the Quit Date, you are no longer a smoker. Period.

The cold turkey method is based on the premise that while it may be uncomfortable and physically challenging to abruptly stop smoking, it is not dangerous, and in the end, it is the simplest way to kick the habit. This method involves no slow weaning off the weed—just a clean, fast break.

HOW DOES IT WORK?

As we discussed on page 10, nicotine, one of the primary chemical components of a cigarette, behaves like candy for the brain by increasing levels of the chemical dopamine, and thus providing feelings of enjoyment. Because the use of nicotine triggers our reward system, we want to use nicotine again and again so we can keep feeling good. This is the addiction-forming aspect of nicotine; the more we use it, the more we want it, and the more we need it to feel good.

The cold turkey method involves cutting the supply of candy to your brain. It is a direct severance, not a slow taper. Stopping the supply abruptly breaks the habit-forming cycle of smoking the cigarette, feeling good, smoking more to keep feeling good, etc.

Of course, in response to the sudden removal of tobacco, the brain triggers withdrawal symptoms such as irritability, frustration, anxiety, restlessness, and insomnia. This is the brain's way of demanding that you provide the drug it needs to feel good.

The withdrawal process can be compared to having a small, whining child nag you to buy a piece of candy for him. The child asks for the candy. You say "no" and explain that the candy is bad for him. The child responds by asking again, and you say "no" again. And the battle of wills continues. What happens if you give in to the child's whining demands? Of course, he stops nagging you . . . for now. But the next time he wants candy, the whining starts all over again. What happens if you consistently refuse to give the child another piece of candy? He stops nagging you about it forever, because he knows that he will not get it.

Similarly, if you say "no" to cigarettes and refuse to take even another puff, your nagging inner voice will eventually stop. Studies show that nicotine withdrawal symptoms peak from twenty-four to forty-eight hours after stopping, and can last—at a lower level—for anywhere from three days to four weeks, with the average being about three weeks. During this time, as you ignore the withdrawal symptoms and refuse to give your body the nicotine it wants, the symptoms become milder and easier to endure. Eventually, your brain stops creating the withdrawal symptoms entirely.

HOW DO YOU USE IT?

In theory, at least, there's no simpler method to use than the cold turkey technique. You just stop smoking.

The night before your Quit Date, throw away all your cigarettes and toss your lighter into the garbage. If the idea appeals to you, make a ceremony out of it and *burn* the cigarettes. You might even want to start a journal to mark the occasion and to serve as an emotional outlet during the quitting process. The point is to get the cigarettes out of your house—and your car and your office—so that they are not within reach when temptation hits.

As I said, the cold turkey method is simple in theory. In practice, however, you will have a better chance of success if you prepare yourself for the

When the Problem Isn't Withdrawal Symptoms

On page 40, you learned that symptoms of withdrawal from tobacco gradually lessen over a period of days, until they disappear. But what if several weeks after you quit smoking, you still feel tense, have difficulty concentrating, or experience other mood or behavior problems? The fact is that what you're experiencing may not be caused by nicotine withdrawal, but may have more to do with emotional disorders such as depression or mania—problems that can become worse once the self-medication provided by smoking is withdrawn. Below, you'll find the most common symptoms of these disorders.

Symptoms of Clinical Depression

- Sadness
- Tension
- Feelings of guilt
- Loss of energy
- Change in appetite
- Inability to concentrate
- Inability to make decisions
- Decreased interest in activities you used to enjoy
- Loss of interest in sex
- Thoughts of hurting or killing yourself

Symptoms of Mania or Bipolar Disorder

- Decreased attention
- Distractibility
- Racing thoughts
- Racing speech
- Inability to sleep
- Rapid mood swings
- Excessive risk-taking
- Spending sprees
- Diminished appetite
- Decreased need for sleep

While none of the above symptoms alone indicates an emotional problem, if you are experiencing several of these symptoms, you may be suffering from a clinical disorder. The good news is that these illnesses can be treated, and that the treatment will not only improve your overall health, but also greatly increase your chance of successfully giving up smoking. If you suspect that you are having emotional problems, contact your physician immediately so that you can get the medical care you need.

task, anticipate possible problems, and have some solutions on hand. Here are some suggestions:

❏ As discussed in Part One (see page 28), you will more effectively use *any* method of quitting if before beginning, you identify your core values. For instance, your core value may be maintaining good health so that you can be an active part of your children's lives, and see them grow up and have children of their own. If you remember this core value and keep it foremost in your mind, it will be all the easier for you to walk past the convenience store without running in for a pack of cigarettes. In fact, you will *have* to walk past it in order to remain true to yourself.

❏ If possible, get help from a stop-smoking program that includes either individual or group counseling. These programs—which provide encouragement and guide you in avoiding common mistakes—can double your chance of success. (See page 34 for more information.)

❏ Tell friends and family members that you have quit, and reach out to them for help when you need it. Some smokers use cigarettes as their support. If this is true of you, now is the time to make a change. I think you'll find that humans make a far better support group than a pack of cigarettes.

❏ If you miss having a cigarette in your mouth, try toothpicks, cinnamon sticks, lollipops or other hard candy, sugar-free gum, or carrot or celery sticks.

❏ If you miss holding a cigarette in your hand, replace it with a pencil, a paper clip, a marble, or a bottle of water.

❏ Keep your hands (and your mind) busy. Do crossword puzzles or needlework; try sketching or painting; clean closets; do woodworking or gardening.

❏ Try to avoid your usual triggers. If you always light up when taking a coffee break with your coworkers, skip your usual break routine and, instead, take a walk or catch up on your reading. If you enjoy a cigarette at the dinner table after your meal, get up from the table as soon as you finish eating. Cigarette smoking is a habit as well as an addiction, and habits can be broken.

❏ When a craving hits, close your eyes and count slowly down from ten to zero, breathing deeply with each count. If that doesn't work, call a friend or take a walk—even if it's just to the end of your driveway. The trick is to find some diversion until the craving passes. And it will.

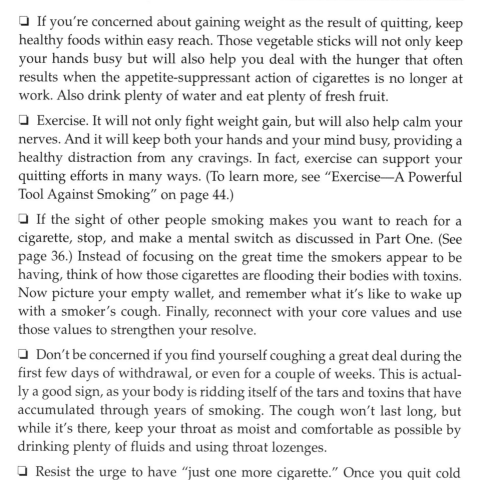

❏ If you're concerned about gaining weight as the result of quitting, keep healthy foods within easy reach. Those vegetable sticks will not only keep your hands busy but will also help you deal with the hunger that often results when the appetite-suppressant action of cigarettes is no longer at work. Also drink plenty of water and eat plenty of fresh fruit.

❏ Exercise. It will not only fight weight gain, but will also help calm your nerves. And it will keep both your hands and your mind busy, providing a healthy distraction from any cravings. In fact, exercise can support your quitting efforts in many ways. (To learn more, see "Exercise—A Powerful Tool Against Smoking" on page 44.)

❏ If the sight of other people smoking makes you want to reach for a cigarette, stop, and make a mental switch as discussed in Part One. (See page 36.) Instead of focusing on the great time the smokers appear to be having, think of how those cigarettes are flooding their bodies with toxins. Now picture your empty wallet, and remember what it's like to wake up with a smoker's cough. Finally, reconnect with your core values and use those values to strengthen your resolve.

❏ Don't be concerned if you find yourself coughing a great deal during the first few days of withdrawal, or even for a couple of weeks. This is actually a good sign, as your body is ridding itself of the tars and toxins that have accumulated through years of smoking. The cough won't last long, but while it's there, keep your throat as moist and comfortable as possible by drinking plenty of fluids and using throat lozenges.

❏ Resist the urge to have "just one more cigarette." Once you quit cold turkey, *you quit.* If you give yourself the option of having another cigarette, you will keep sliding. And every time you give in, you will have to start at the beginning again. Don't do that to yourself. Once you've made the commitment to quit, keep your commitment.

In addition to using the above tips, remember that any withdrawal symptoms you're feeling will lessen as you continue to live smoke-free. The trick is to hang in there and, when cravings get bad, to access your core values. Novelist William Faulkner said, "The man who removes a mountain begins by carrying away small stones." Similarly, you will quit for first a minute at a time, then an hour at a time. Those minutes and hours will add up until you find that it's been weeks since your last smoke. And some day, you'll realize that it's been years since you had a cigarette.

Exercise—A Powerful Tool Against Smoking

You already know that exercise offers an array of benefits, ranging from better overall health to a reduced risk of heart attack and stroke. But did you know that it can also help you stop smoking?

Exercise supports the effort to quit smoking in a variety of ways. First, it's a distraction. You can get lost in exercise just as you can get lost in a good book or an engrossing movie. And when you're focused on exercise, you're *not* focused on smoking. In fact, assuming that you've been given clearance by your doctor (more on that later), you can exercise any nicotine cravings right out of your body by going for a run!

Second, exercise can be used as a form of meditation. At some point during exercise, your concentration is focused intently on your breathing, the pounding of your feet, or the movement of a ball—depending, of course, on the specific exercise you're doing. You stop thinking; you stop worrying about the day's events. The stresses in your life melt away. When you emerge from your exercise session, you may feel as if you've been on a brief vacation. As you reenter your world, you do so with a relaxed mind and body, and a fresh perspective.

Third, exercise has been shown to alter hormone levels in a way that has a positive effect on mood. For this reason, exercise can directly help you fight withdrawal symptoms such as anxiety and irritability.

Fourth, as mentioned on page 43, exercise can help you combat the weight gain that many people associate with giving up cigarettes. This can help you stick with your commitment to quit.

Finally, like quitting smoking, beginning an exercise program is an important lifestyle change. So exercise can reinforce your commitment to making positive changes in the way you live. In a sense, you will be replacing the deadly habit of smoking with the life-affirming habit of exercising.

Of course, if you haven't exercised for years, it is vital that you talk to your doctor before starting an exercise program. While exercise can be healthful, it can also be dangerous, depending on your physical condition and on the type of activity you choose. Only your physician can evaluate your health and help you select an exercise regimen that is safe, and that will provide you with the benefits you want.

Once your doctor has given you the go-ahead, you'll want to choose a form of exercise and begin making it a habit. Here are some tips:

❏ If you are a former athlete who hasn't exercised in years, don't think that you can do what you used to do. You can't—or, at least, you can't without incurring injury. Be sure to start gradually, and to diligently stretch your muscles before and after every exercise session. In fact, any exercise should start with a ten- to fifteen-minute warm-up, and end with a ten- to fifteen-minute cool-down.

❏ Select an exercise you enjoy. If you love the outdoors, consider running or bicycling. If you love being around people, consider joining a gym. If you enjoy watching TV, set up a TV in front of your treadmill or elliptical machine, or select a gym that has television sets at each workout station. If you love to dance, find a local dance class. As soon as you get bored with your exercise routine, you'll quit, so pick an activity you think you'll enjoy, and "tweak" it as necessary to keep it interesting.

❏ If possible, start an exercise program under the supervision of a personal trainer. A good trainer can help you design an appropriate and effective exercise program, can be motivational, and can help you avoid injury. Just be sure to choose a trainer as you would select any professional. Do your research, check his or her credentials, and if possible, get a referral from a doctor or a friend. And if you can't hire a trainer, consider attending a supervised class, where the leader can give you suggestions and tips.

❏ Get an exercise buddy. You'll be more likely to go out running or drive to the gym if you'll be joining a friend once you get there.

❏ Make exercise a habit. You wouldn't go through the day without brushing your teeth, would you? Exercise has to become as automatic as tooth brushing. To turn it into a habit, you'll need to be consistent, especially during the first few weeks. Ideally, you should exercise for thirty to sixty minutes, five to six times per week.

Remember that the benefits of exercise have as much to do with the process as they do with the end result. Although the destination—a healthier, stronger, smoke-free body—is highly desirable, you have to enjoy the trip, as well. That way, you'll be sure to make exercise an important part of your life.

HOW WELL DOES IT WORK?

Smoking is an addiction, and the addiction is different for every person. For that reason, the withdrawal process is more difficult for some smokers than it is for others. And, of course, some people approach the cold turkey method with more resolve than others.

About 25 percent of those who quit cold turkey return to smoking after only forty-eight hours, and the relapse rate rises to 60 percent two weeks after the Quit Date. A year later, only a small percentage are still nonsmokers. Nevertheless, studies have shown that an amazingly high percentage of former smokers—*over 90 percent,* according to the American Cancer Society—quit smoking cold turkey. So while many people may fail to quit at any given time, over the years, many have succeeded using the cold turkey method. Remember: Most successful quitters, quit and relapse several times before giving up smoking for good.

Certainly, quitting cold turkey isn't easy. But your temperament, the level of your addiction, and the number of times you have tried to quit before will all play a role in determining if it works for you. Just about all of us know someone who has successfully quit smoking cold turkey.

The Pros and Cons of Cold Turkey

The Pros

❏ You can use it any time.

❏ It's free.

❏ It involves no drugs, and can be used regardless of any medical problems you have and any medications you may be using.

❏ No prescription or over-the-counter aid is needed.

The Cons

❏ It doesn't help you cope with withdrawal symptoms or cravings.

❏ It provides no cigarette substitute—nothing to hold in your hand or place in your mouth.

RISKS AND DISADVANTAGES

Unlike the withdrawal from other drugs, such as alcohol, nicotine withdrawal poses no direct risk to your health. For that reason, although the cold turkey method will likely result in withdrawal symptoms, it is not at all dangerous.

Of course, the disadvantage of cold turkey quitting is that the system offers no help or support through medications or other forms of aid. While many people are able to successfully quit without assistance, others find the withdrawal symptoms too distressing and the cravings too tempting. These people might benefit from further quit-smoking tools.

CONCLUSION

Cold turkey quitting is available to everyone. It's free, and it doesn't require a doctor's appointment, a prescription, or a trip to your local acupuncturist. Moreover, you can use this technique at any time simply by making the decision to quit.

Is cold turkey right for you? The only way to find out is to try it. But before you do, it makes sense to consider the other options presented in this book. Remember that for many people, a combination of techniques provides the best solution. For example, you can pair the cold turkey method with nicotine replacement therapy, hypnosis, or another technique that will help you minimize withdrawal symptoms and maintain motivation. The fact is that a lot of help is readily available. It's up to you to find the method or combination of methods that works.

#2

Tapering Off

While many people try to stop smoking using the cold turkey method described in the previous chapter, many others attempt to quit more gradually by slowly decreasing the number of cigarettes they smoke each day. Tapering off has the same result as quitting cold turkey, but is done at your own pace. You are the driver who gauges the speed at which you give up smoking.

Like quitting cold turkey, the tapering method is free, and can be used without a prescription drug or other aid. Plus, the fact that it's gradual appeals to many people, as it allows more time to both emotionally and physically adjust to life without cigarettes. Would it work for you? That's what this chapter is all about.

WHAT IS IT?

Like cold turkey quitting, tapering off involves picking a Quit Date. However, in this case, you also set up a schedule that details the number of cigarettes you will smoke each day *prior* to the Quit Date. Then, following the schedule, you gradually decrease your cigarette use. When you reach your Quit Date, you are no longer a smoker.

The tapering off method is based on the premise that it is easier to slowly wean yourself off smoking than it is to abruptly quit. By gradually decreasing the number of cigarettes you use each day, you may make your withdrawal symptoms less severe and easier to endure.

HOW DOES IT WORK?

Earlier in the book, you learned that the nicotine in cigarettes provides feelings of enjoyment by increasing levels of the chemical dopamine in the brain. But nicotine does more than produce a feeling of pleasure. It creates an addiction that causes your brain to punish you when smoking stops. As long as you keep the nicotine streaming in, the feelings of enjoyment continue. But when the supply of tobacco is severed, you experience symptoms such as irritability, frustration, anxiety, restlessness, and insomnia.

As you might expect, when the supply of cigarettes is severed all at once, withdrawal symptoms can be harsh—although the severity of symptoms varies from person to person. That's why many people feel more comfortable using the tapering method, which allows the brain to become used to gradually decreasing amounts of nicotine. It is thought that this results in relatively mild symptoms that continue to lessen in severity until they disappear altogether. The tapering method also gives you more time to say good-bye to cigarettes and make the mental adjustments needed to accept a smoke-free lifestyle.

HOW DO YOU USE IT?

The tapering off method is a bit more complicated than going cold turkey. You still choose a Quit Date, but this time, you also create a schedule that details the number of cigarettes you will smoke each day prior to the Quit Date, with the amount gradually decreasing as time goes on.

There is no special formula for tapering. The schedule you use is your decision, and will be at least partly based on the number of cigarettes you now smoke on a daily basis. Let's say, for example, that you now smoke a pack each day, or twenty cigarettes. You may want to choose a tapering schedule in which you smoke twenty cigarettes on day one, nineteen on day two, eighteen on day three, and so on, decreasing the amount by one cigarette each day. Or you may feel more comfortable smoking twenty cigarettes on day one, eighteen on days two through seven, sixteen on days eight through sixteen, and so on, until you reach your Quit Date. You can even taper more gradually by smoking twenty cigarettes for the first two weeks, eighteen for the next two weeks, etc. The possibilities are endless.

Once you've decided on your schedule, use a calendar to record exactly how many cigarettes you are allotted each day, and on which day you will smoke no cigarettes at all. If your plan isn't down on paper—and especially if you just have a loose agreement with yourself to "gradually cut down"—you'll make it too easy to slide. Cutting down is great, but if you want to quit smoking, you have to create a precise schedule, write it down, and stick to it.

While the tapering off method may seem cut-and-dried—after all, you're simply following a schedule—you will have a greater chance of success if you keep some simple guidelines in mind. Also, although your withdrawal symptoms may be milder than they would if you were quitting cold turkey, realize that you're still going to have them, along with cravings. That's why it's important to anticipate possible problems and have some proven solutions at your fingertips. Here are some tips:

❏ As discussed in Part One (see page 28), you will more effectively use *any* method of quitting if before beginning, you identify your core values. For instance, your core value may be maintaining good health so that you enjoy a long and active retirement with your spouse. If you remember this core value and keep it foremost in your mind, it will be all the easier for you to stick to your schedule until you reach your Quit Date.

❏ If possible, get help from a stop-smoking program that includes either individual or group counseling. These programs—which provide encouragement and guide you in avoiding common mistakes—can double your chance of success. (See page 34 for more information.)

❏ Tell friends and family members that you have quit, and reach out to them for help when you need it. Some smokers use cigarettes as their support. If this is true of you, now is the time to make a change. I think you'll find that humans make a far better support group than a pack of cigarettes.

❏ Try to design your schedule so by your Quit Date, you are smoking no more than half as many cigarettes as you were smoking prior to using the tapering method. The less you are smoking by your Quit Date, the better.

❏ Each day, carry with you only the number of cigarettes you've allotted for that day. Carrying a full pack of cigarettes on a day when you're allowed ten is a sure recipe for failure.

❏ If you have smoked your limit for the day, and you miss having a cigarette in your mouth, try toothpicks, cinnamon sticks, lollipops or other hard candy, sugar-free gum, or carrot or celery sticks.

❏ If you miss holding a cigarette in your hand, replace it with a pencil, a paper clip, a marble, or a bottle of water.

❏ Keep your hands (and your mind) busy. Do crossword puzzles or needlework; try sketching or painting; clean closets; do woodworking or gardening.

❏ Once you've smoked your limit for the day, try to avoid your usual triggers. If you always light up when taking a coffee break with your coworkers, skip your usual break routine and, instead, take a walk or catch up on your reading. If you enjoy a cigarette at the dinner table after your meal, get up from the table as soon as you finish eating. Cigarette smoking is a habit as well as an addiction, and habits can be broken.

❏ If a craving hits, and you've already smoked that day's limit, close your eyes and count slowly down from ten to zero, breathing deeply with each count. If that doesn't work, call a friend or take a walk—even if it's just to the end of your driveway. The trick is to find some diversion until the craving passes. And it will.

❏ If you're concerned about gaining weight as the result of quitting, keep healthy foods within easy reach. Those vegetable sticks will not only keep your hands busy but will also help you deal with the hunger that often results when the appetite-suppressant action of cigarettes is no longer at work. Also drink plenty of water and eat plenty of fresh fruit.

❏ Exercise. It will not only fight weight gain, but will also help calm your nerves. And it will keep both your hands and your mind busy, providing a healthy distraction from any cravings. In fact, exercise can support your quit-smoking efforts in many ways. (To learn more, see "Exercise—A Powerful Tool Against Smoking" on page 44.)

❏ If the sight of other people smoking makes you want to reach for a cigarette, and you've already had your limit, make a mental switch, as discussed in Part One. (See page 36.) Instead of focusing on the great time the smokers appear to be having, think of how those cigarettes are flooding their bodies with toxins. Now picture your empty wallet, and remember what it's like to wake up with a smoker's cough. Finally, reconnect with your core values and use those values to strengthen your resolve.

❏ Don't be concerned if you find yourself coughing a great deal as you slowly cut down on your smoking, or even after your Quit Date. This is actually a good sign, as your body is ridding itself of the tars and toxins that have accumulated through years of smoking. The cough won't last long, but while it's there, keep your throat as moist and comfortable as possible by drinking plenty of fluids and using throat lozenges.

❏ Resist the urge to have "just one more cigarette." Once you've had your day's limit, don't give yourself the option of having another cigarette, or you will keep sliding. Similarly, don't "reward" yourself with more cigarettes after successfully tapering for a few days. If you want this method to work, your schedule must be unidirectional. In other words, you must gradually and continually decrease the number of cigarettes smoked, without allowing yourself any increases. Remember the reason for tapering off: You're trying to get your brain used to gradually decreasing levels of nicotine. If you lessen the amount of nicotine only to increase it again, the method won't work.

In addition to using the above tips and guidelines, remember that any withdrawal symptoms you feel, whether severe or mild, will lessen as your body gradually becomes accustomed to lower amounts of nicotine, and finally is cut off from cigarettes entirely. In the meantime, you have to hang in there, stick to your schedule, and when cravings or withdrawal symptoms get bad, access your core values. Try not to look ahead when following your schedule. Take it one day at a time, sticking to your cigarette allotment for that day. Gradually, you will realize that you have been sticking to the schedule for days, and then for weeks, until you are finally free of cigarettes.

HOW WELL DOES IT WORK?

Smoking is an addiction, and the addiction is different for every person. For that reason, the withdrawal process is more difficult for some smokers than it is for other. And, of course, some people approach the tapering method with strong resolve, while others—whether consciously or unconsciously—use it as an excuse to put off quitting.

In the previous chapter, you learned that most people who quit, quit cold turkey. There is evidence that the slower, "gentler" tapering method is not as effective as the cold turkey technique. But if this is the right method for you—if you need to temper the withdrawal symptoms through gradual tapering, but have the discipline it takes to adhere to a schedule—it really doesn't matter what the studies indicate. The fact is that many people quit smoking by tapering off.

RISKS AND DISADVANTAGES

Like quitting cold turkey, the tapering method poses no risks to your health simply because nicotine withdrawal poses no risk to your health. Yes, you will probably experience withdrawal symptoms using this method, but they will not be dangerous.

On the other hand, many people feel that tapering has several disadvantages. The first is one shared with the cold turkey technique: The tapering method offers no help or support through medications or other forms of aid. For some people, the nature of this technique makes the withdrawal symptoms relatively mild so that no help is needed from pills, patches, or other quit-smoking tools. But others find the withdrawal symptoms too distressing and the cravings too tempting.

Some people also feel that the tapering method merely prolongs discomfort. They liken it to pulling off a bandage slowly and torturously, rather than briskly ripping it off. Either way, you're going to feel discomfort, but would you rather feel it all at once, or endure a lesser degree of pain for a longer period of time? Only you can answer that question.

Some smokers say that as soon as they put a cigarette in their mouth, they begin to crave the next. For them, each cigarette increases the desire to smoke and continues the cycle of addiction. If this is true of you, a slow,

The Pros and Cons of Tapering Off

The Pros

❏ You can use it any time.

❏ It's free.

❏ It involves no drugs, and can be used regardless of any medical problems you have and any medications you may be taking.

❏ No prescription or over-the-counter aid is needed.

The Cons

❏ It doesn't help you cope with withdrawal symptoms or cravings.

❏ The cigarettes allowed while tapering actually *increase* cravings for some people.

❏ Some people inhale very deeply when smoking their allotted cigarettes, temporarily increasing blood carbon monoxide levels.

gradual withdrawal may be impossible. Instead, quitting must be an all-or-nothing proposition.

The tapering method has one more disadvantage. Some people find that since they are allotted only so many cigarettes per day, when they do smoke, they inhale harder and deeper. Although the method still may work, be aware that this habit results in a temporary (although not dangerous) increase in blood carbon monoxide levels.

CONCLUSION

Like quitting cold turkey, quitting through gradual tapering is available to everyone. Armed with resolve, a calendar, and a pencil, you can draw up a plan and start moving toward a smoke-free life today.

Is tapering right for you? Now that you know the pros and cons of this method, you may be able to answer this question. Can you put together a realistic plan and stick to it? Will smoking several cigarettes every day make the quitting process easier for you, or more difficult?

Perhaps you can discover if tapering is right for you only by trying it out. But before you pull out your calendar and start jotting down your schedule, it may make sense to consider the other options presented in this book. Studies have shown that for many people, a combination of techniques is needed for success. You might, for instance, combine tapering with hypnosis. An added quit-smoking method could further temper your withdrawal symptoms, help keep both your spirits and your motivation high during the tapering process and beyond, and ultimately enable you to live a smoke-free lifestyle.

#3

The Nicotine Patch

The previous two chapters discussed quitting methods that essentially rely on willpower to cope with withdrawal symptoms and cravings. But the fact is that the physical symptoms caused by nicotine withdrawal are one of the primary reasons that people return to smoking. Willpower isn't always enough.

Nicotine replacement therapy (NRT) was designed to reduce withdrawal symptoms by supplying a relatively safe source of nicotine in measured doses that can be decreased in strength, until the supply of nicotine is completely stopped. This therapy has helped many people successfully stop smoking.

Several types of NRT are now on the market. Nicotine patches, gum, and lozenges are available without a prescription, while nicotine nasal sprays and inhalers are available through prescription only. This chapter will examine the nicotine patch so that you can decide if it would help you in your efforts to quit smoking. In later chapters, you'll learn about other forms of nicotine replacement therapy.

WHAT IS IT?

The nicotine patch looks like a large adhesive bandage, with an outer rim that sticks to the skin, and an inner area that presses against the skin, slowly releasing nicotine into the body. The patch comes in several different strengths—such as 7, 14, and 21 milligrams—so that smokers can use the strength that is appropriate for both their body weight and the amount of nicotine they are used to getting from cigarettes. (The average cigarette delivers roughly 2 milligrams of nicotine, with some containing less and some containing more.) Kits generally supply a sufficient number of patches to last through the process of quitting.

The patch is intended to be worn either sixteen or twenty-four hours a day, depending on the type chosen, and replaced at the same time each day. By continuously delivering nicotine into the system, it prevents or reduces the withdrawal symptoms that usually result from smoking cessation, making it easier to quit smoking.

HOW DOES IT WORK?

As you learned earlier in the book, the nicotine in cigarettes provides feelings of enjoyment by increasing brain levels of the chemical dopamine—a substance associated with the pleasure system of the brain. As nicotine creates a feeling of pleasure time and time again, it also creates an addiction that causes your brain to punish you when smoking stops. When the supply of tobacco is severed, you experience symptoms such as irritability, frustration, anxiety, restlessness, and insomnia. Many people find these symptoms so distressing that they start smoking cigarettes again despite their desire to quit.

The nicotine patch helps you stop smoking by bringing nicotine into your body via a different delivery system—a safer delivery system that does not provide the tars, carbon monoxide, and other toxic chemicals contained in cigarettes. Because your brain is not starved of nicotine, it produces either no withdrawal symptoms or less severe symptoms, making it easier to quit.

It's important to understand that all NRTs work in different ways, and that the patch is the only NRT that does not simulate the highs and lows of nicotine normally experienced while smoking cigarettes. Instead, throughout the day, it delivers a slow, constant, low level of nicotine.

HOW DO YOU USE IT?

The nicotine patch must be used in combination with cold turkey quitting. You cannot smoke while using the patch, as this can result in an overdose of nicotine. For that reason, your first step in using this technique is to choose a Quit Date, just as you would if you were quitting cold turkey without the help of an NRT.

Next, you must choose the right strength patch. Since the best strength depends on both your body weight and the amount of cigarettes you smoke each day, it would be a good idea to speak to your physician or pharmacist before buying the patch. Also consider whether you want a twenty-four-hour or sixteen-hour patch. If your morning cravings for cigarettes are severe, a twenty-four-hour patch may be your best bet. Be aware, though, that the twenty-four-hour patch can cause sleep disturbances, such as insomnia or unusually vivid dreams. For this reason, some people start with the twenty-four-hour patch and then switch to a sixteen-hour type.

When your Quit Date arrives and you stop smoking, each day, you must place a new patch on a clean, dry, hairless patch of skin between your neck and waist. The upper arm or shoulder is often a good choice, but you can also apply it to your stomach or side. The patch should never be cut into smaller pieces, and must be removed from its wrapper right before application. Of course, each patch should be worn only for the number of hours specified, whether sixteen or twenty-four.

Follow the manufacturer's directions regarding the number of weeks you stay on the patch. With some brands, you use patches at one strength for four weeks, taper down to lower-strength patches for another four weeks, and then stop using the patch entirely. Some brands supply enough patches for ten weeks; some, for a longer period of time. If you think you may need or want to use the patch for longer than six months, be sure to consult a doctor.

Although the nicotine patch can help you quit smoking, it's important to understand that the patch alone will not enable you to give up cigarettes. Smokers are addicted not just to nicotine, but to the entire smoking experience. For that reason, you'll have greatest success using the patch if you anticipate possible problems and have some solutions on hand. Note, too, that because the patch delivers a drug into your system, you'll want to take certain precautions to make the quitting experience as safe as possible. These tips should help:

❑ As discussed in Part One (see page 28), you will more effectively use *any* method of quitting if before beginning, you identify your core values. For instance, your core value may be maintaining good health so that you can be an active part of your children's lives, and see them grow up and have children of their own. If you remember this core value and keep it foremost in your mind, it will be all the easier for you to keep away from cigarettes.

❑ If possible, get help from a stop-smoking program that includes either individual or group counseling. These programs—which provide encouragement and guide you in avoiding common mistakes—can double your chance of success. (See page 34 for more information.)

❏ Tell friends and family members that you have quit, and reach out to them for help when you need it. Some smokers use cigarettes as their support. If this is true of you, now is the time to make a change. I think you'll find that humans make a far better support group than a pack of cigarettes.

❏ If you miss having a cigarette in your mouth, try toothpicks, cinnamon sticks, lollipops or other hard candy, sugar-free gum, or carrot or celery sticks.

❏ If you miss holding a cigarette in your hand, replace it with a pencil, a paper clip, a marble, or a bottle of water.

❏ Keep your hands (and your mind) busy. Do crossword puzzles or needlework; try sketching or painting; clean closets; do woodworking or gardening.

❏ Try to avoid your usual triggers. If you always light up when taking a coffee break with your coworkers, skip your usual break routine and, instead, take a walk or catch up on your reading. If you enjoy a cigarette at the dinner table after your meal, get up from the table as soon as you finish eating. Cigarette smoking is a habit as well as an addiction, and habits can be broken.

❏ When a craving hits, close your eyes and count slowly down from ten to zero, breathing deeply with each count. If that doesn't work, call a friend or take a walk—even if it's just to the end of your driveway. The trick is to find some diversion until the craving passes. And it will.

❏ If you're concerned about gaining weight as the result of quitting, keep healthy foods within easy reach. Those vegetable sticks will not only keep your hands busy but will also help you deal with the hunger that often results when the appetite-suppressant action of cigarettes is no longer at work. Also drink plenty of water and eat plenty of fresh fruit.

❏ Exercise. It will not only fight weight gain, but will also keep both your hands and your mind busy, providing a healthy distraction from any cravings. In fact, exercise can support your quit-smoking efforts in many ways. (To learn more, see "Exercise—A Powerful Tool Against Smoking" on page 44.)

❏ If the sight of other people smoking makes you want to reach for a cigarette, stop, and make a mental switch as discussed in Part One. (See page 36.) Instead of focusing on the great time the smokers appear to be having, think of how those cigarettes are flooding their bodies with toxins. Now picture your empty wallet, and remember what it's like to wake up with a smoker's cough. Finally, reconnect with your core values and use those values to strengthen your resolve.

❏ Don't be concerned if you find yourself coughing after you begin use of the patch. Although the patch lessens the severity of withdrawal symptoms, you may still cough as your body rids itself of the tars and toxins that have accumulated through years of smoking. Accept this as a good sign— a sign of healing—and keep your throat as moist and comfortable as possible by drinking plenty of fluids and using throat lozenges.

❏ Resist the urge to have "just one more cigarette." Once you quit cold turkey, *you quit.* More important, using any NRT and smoking at the same time is dangerous because it can cause you to overdose on nicotine.

❏ Do not try to make quitting easier by using multiple forms of NRT, such as both the patch and nicotine gum, without medical supervision. This, too, can result in nicotine overdose. Use a combination of these tools only under the guidance of your doctor. (See "Can You Use More Than One NRT At a Time?" on page 63.)

❏ If you find yourself overwhelmed by cravings for nicotine, don't add another patch to the first one, but consider switching to a stronger patch. If you are already wearing the strongest patch, consider the possibility that the patch might not right for you. You may need another type of NRT, or you may need an entirely different type of quit-smoking tool.

❏ Wear the patch for the number of hours specified by the manufacturer, rather than putting it on intermittently as a substitute for cigarette smoking. If an intermittent dose of nicotine is what you need, you should be using nicotine gum or lozenges. Similarly, do not remove the patch in order to smoke, and then slap it back on when your cigarette break is over. This will defeat the purpose of using the NRT.

❏ To avoid skin irritation, rotate patch locations rather than applying patches to the same area, day after day. You should generally wait a week before re-using an area. Also be sure to wash your hands after putting on the patch. Any nicotine that gets on your hands can be transferred to your eyes or nose and cause problems such as stinging.

❑ Keep the patch (whether new or used) away from children and pets, and do not use the patch if you are pregnant or nursing unless your doctor directs you to do so. Again, it's important to remember that the patch is a drug, and must be used with caution.

Keep in mind that even when using the patch, quitting will require iron resolve. NRTs do not eliminate your emotional attachment to cigarettes. And NRTs usually don't replace the full amount of nicotine you've been getting from cigarettes, so you may still have some mild withdrawal symptoms. Don't expect quitting to be a walk in the park just because you're using the patch. But if you're determined to quit and you want to temper possible withdrawal symptoms, the patch may be the answer. Of all the NRTs now available, it is the most convenient to use and the most inconspicuous, as well. Once you apply it, it remains in place under your clothing, working for you all day.

HOW WELL DOES IT WORK?

Smoking is an addiction, and the addiction is different for every person. For that reason, the withdrawal process is more difficult for some smokers than it is for others even when the patch is in use. But evidence shows that the patch can be effective. According to studies, 25 to 30 percent of people who use some form of nicotine replacement therapy are smoke-free six months after starting use of the NRT. After a year, NRTs appears to be about twice as effective as quitting cold turkey without any aids. Note that the patch has been found to be neither more nor less effective than nicotine lozenges and gum. The rate of success appears to be the same for these three forms of NRT.

RISKS AND DISADVANTAGES

To start, it's important to understand that using any nicotine replacement therapy, including the patch, is much safer for you than smoking cigarettes. Remember that cigarettes contain thousands of toxic chemicals, while an NRT supplies only nicotine.

With that said, it's impossible to overemphasize the fact that the nicotine patch is a drug, and that it must be used with caution. It's a good idea to discuss the patch with your doctor before purchasing it. He or she can guide you in choosing the best patch for your needs, and help monitor any

Can You Use More Than One NRT At a Time?

Some smokers feel that if one NRT is good, several are even better. So on their own—with the idea of preventing any and all withdrawal symptoms—they wear the patch, chew the gum, and maybe even suck on a nicotine lozenge now and then.

As mentioned on page 61, you should *not* combine several forms of NRT on your own, as this can lead to a dangerous overdose of nicotine. But if you feel that you need more help than the patch provides, by all means speak to your doctor about the judicious use of two types of nicotine replacement therapy. You may, for instance, use the patch to provide a continual low level of nicotine delivery, and then chew nicotine gum once in a while to deal with breakthrough withdrawal symptoms. As the weeks go by, you will taper down the use of both the gum and the patch, until you are free of nicotine.

Yes, the use of two types of NRT can help keep withdrawal symptoms at bay. Just be sure to get your doctor's okay, and to use these powerful quit-smoking tools exactly as your physician directs.

problems throughout the quitting process. Moreover, if your physician prescribes the NRT, your health insurance may actually cover it, making it more affordable.

Most important, though, you must confer with your doctor if you are pregnant, planning to become pregnant, or nursing; if you are under the age of eighteen; or if you have one of the following conditions:

- Asthma
- Atopic dermatitis
- Cardiovascular disease, including angina pectoris (chest pain), arrhythmia, and recent heart attack
- Diabetes
- Eczema
- High blood pressure
- Impaired circulation
- Kidney disease
- Liver disease

- Lung disease, such as emphysema

- Pheochromocytoma (a tumor of the adrenal gland)

- Psoriasis

- Recurrent nasal allergies

- Stomach ulcer

- Thyroid problems

Although one or more of the above conditions won't necessarily rule out use of the patch, they may make it necessary for your doctor to recommend a product that's a better match for your individual risk profile. For instance, if you have eczema, psoriasis, or another skin condition, the patch may be a poor choice as it may exacerbate your existing problem. In such a case, your doctor may suggest a different NRT, or another type of quit-smoking aid entirely. In the case of heart disease, nicotine replacement therapy may not be the treatment of choice because nicotine can actually increase the heart's workload by raising heart rate and blood pressure. On the other hand, your doctor may feel that in your case, the patch poses a far lesser risk than that of continued smoking.

When discussing the possible use of an NRT with your doctor, be sure to mention all the medications you're currently taking, including prescription drugs and over-the-counter medications. Especially tell your doctor if you are taking one of the following:

- Acetaminophen (Tylenol and others)

- Caffeine

- Diuretics (water pills)

- Imipramine (Tofranil, Janimine)

- Insulin

- High blood pressure medications

- Oxazepam (Serax)

- Pentazocine (Talwin, Talwin NX, Talacen)

- Propoxyphene (Darvon, Darvon-N, E-Lor, PC-CAP, Wygesic, and others)

- Propranolol (Inderal)

- Theophylline (Aerolate, Asmalix, Theo-Dur, and others)
- Vitamins

Again, use of any of the above substances may not rule out use of the patch. But in some cases, your doctor may suggest a different quit-smoking technique.

Earlier, I mentioned that the patch can cause unpleasant, disruptive dreams. Other possible side effects include the following:

- Abdominal pain
- Blurred vision
- Diarrhea or upset stomach
- Dizziness
- Headaches
- High blood pressure
- Insomnia
- Itching, burning, redness, or swelling at application site
- Nausea and/or vomiting
- Weakness

By rotating the site of application, you may be able to avoid or eliminate problems such as redness and swelling. Switching brands can also help. If not, or if you experience any of the other symptoms listed above, you should contact your physician to determine if it is safe for you to continue using the patch. Contact your physician *immediately* if you have any of the following problems, which may be signs of nicotine overdose.

- Abnormal heartbeat or rhythm
- Cold sweats
- Difficulty breathing
- Seizures
- Severe abdominal pain
- Severe rash or swelling
- Severe tremors

The lists of potential side effects presented above are not meant to scare you, but to make you aware of the possible consequences of nicotine use or overdose so that you will be alert to problems. Similarly, it's important to understand fully that *you should not smoke when using the patch, or any other NRT.* This can cause a serious nicotine overdose, which can result in death.

In addition to being aware of the potential side effects associated with NRTs in general, it makes sense to understand some drawbacks related specifically to the patch. The first possible drawback is that the patch provides the body with a constant low level of nicotine. While this helps to keep withdrawal symptoms under control, it does not approximate the ups and downs of smoking. For some people, this is a problem. If you think you would actually feel more comfortable with an aid that provides the roller coaster effect of smoking, you might do better with another form of NRT.

The Pros and Cons of the Nicotine Patch

The Pros

❏ It's available over-the-counter.

❏ It lessens withdrawal symptoms and cravings through a continuous supply of nicotine.

❏ It's easy to use; once you put it in place, it works all day.

❏ It's inconspicuous.

❏ If you get a prescription from your doctor, it may be covered by your insurance.

The Cons

❏ It must be purchased.

❏ Because it's a drug, people with certain medical problems cannot use it.

❏ It must be used carefully, and can cause side effects.

❏ It provides no cigarette substitute—nothing to hold in your hand or place in your mouth.

❏ It doesn't provide the highs and lows experienced when getting nicotine from cigarettes.

Another possible problem is that the patch doesn't give you anything to do with your hands or mouth. If you miss holding a cigarette in your hand or putting one in your mouth, again, nicotine gum or lozenges may be a better choice. Some smokers prefer the nicotine inhaler specifically because it simulates the action of putting a cigarette in your mouth.

CONCLUSION

The patch is a readily available over-the-counter aid that can help you quit smoking cold turkey by reducing or eliminating your withdrawal symptoms. Despite the patch's possible side effects, many people have already used this type of nicotine replacement therapy safely. In fact, less than 5 percent of the people who try the patch have to stop use due to side effects. And as mentioned earlier, studies show that the patch can actually *double* your chance of successfully quitting the smoking habit.

Just keep in mind that like any aid, the patch will be effective only if you pair it with motivation and willpower. No form of nicotine replacement therapy can quit smoking for you, but if you access your core values and cement your motivation before your Quit Date, the patch can certainly help you get through the quitting process.

Remember, too, that although the nicotine patch is one of the best known quit-smoking aids, it is not the only aid. For that reason, before settling on the patch, you may want to consider some of the other options available. Perhaps you would have more success if you used another type of NRT, such as nicotine gum or lozenges. Or perhaps you can maximize your success by using the patch along with another tool, such as hypnosis. In the following chapters, you'll learn about other quit-smoking aids that can help you as you move towards a smoke-free lifestyle.

#4

Nicotine Gum

Some quitting methods, like cold turkey and tapering, essentially rely on willpower to cope with withdrawal symptoms and cravings. But the fact is that the physical symptoms caused by nicotine withdrawal are one of the primary reasons that people return to smoking. Willpower isn't always enough.

Nicotine replacement therapy (NRT), which was first discussed in the previous chapter, was designed to reduce withdrawal symptoms by supplying a relatively safe source of nicotine in measured doses that can be reduced in strength or frequency until the supply of nicotine is completely stopped. This therapy has helped many people successfully stop smoking.

Several types of NRT are now on the market. Nicotine patches, gum, and lozenges are available without a prescription, while nicotine nasal sprays and inhalers are available through prescription only. The previous chapter discussed the patch. This chapter will examine nicotine gum so that you can decide if it would help you in your efforts to quit smoking. In later chapters, you'll learn about the remaining forms of nicotine replacement therapy.

WHAT IS IT?

Nicotine chewing gum is a resin complex of nicotine and polacrilin in a sugar-free chewing gum base. The gum includes buffering agents such as sodium carbonate and sodium bicarbonate to increase the pH of the saliva, enhancing the body's absorption of nicotine.

Nicotine gum comes in different strengths—2 milligrams and 4 milligrams—so that smokers can use the strength that is appropriate for the amount of nicotine they are used to getting from cigarettes. (The average cigarette delivers roughly 2 milligrams of nicotine, with some containing less and some containing more.) The gum also is available in different flavors, such as mint and fruit.

This type of NRT is intended to be used either on a regular basis, to prevent or minimize withdrawal symptoms; *or* to stop cravings as they arise.

HOW DOES IT WORK?

As you learned earlier in the book, the nicotine in cigarettes provides feelings of enjoyment by increasing brain levels of the chemical dopamine—a substance associated with the pleasure system of the brain. As nicotine creates a feeling of pleasure time and time again, it also creates an addiction that causes your brain to punish you when smoking stops. When the supply of tobacco is severed, you experience symptoms such as irritability, frustration, anxiety, restlessness, and insomnia. Many people find these symptoms so distressing that they start smoking cigarettes again despite their desire to quit.

Nicotine gum helps you stop smoking by bringing nicotine into your body via a different delivery system—a safer delivery system that does not provide the tars, carbon monoxide, and other toxic chemicals contained in cigarettes. When you chew the gum, the nicotine is released. When you "park" the gum—that is, when you put the gum between your cheek and gums and hold it there—the nicotine is absorbed through the mucous membranes of your mouth into your bloodstream. Because your brain is not starved of nicotine, it produces either no withdrawal symptoms or less severe symptoms, making it easier to quit.

It's important to understand that all NRTs work in different ways. The patch, discussed in the previous chapter, delivers a slow, constant, low level of nicotine. Nicotine gum, however, delivers a measured dose of nicotine only when a piece is chewed. This not only helps simulate the highs and lows of nicotine normally experienced when smoking cigarettes, but also acts as a substitute oral activity.

HOW DO YOU USE IT?

Nicotine gum must be used in combination with cold turkey quitting. You cannot smoke while using the gum, as this can result in an overdose of nicotine. For that reason, your first step in using this technique is to choose a Quit Date, just as you would if you were quitting cold turkey without the help of an NRT.

Next, you must choose the right strength gum—a decision that, for the most part, is based on the number of cigarettes you smoke each day. It is a good idea to speak to your physician or pharmacist regarding the best strength to use. Generally, if you smoke fewer than twenty-five cigarettes a day, you should choose the 2-milligram gum. If you smoke twenty-five or more cigarettes per day, the 4-milligram gum would be a better choice.

When your Quit Date arrives and you stop smoking, you can begin using the nicotine gum to prevent and/or cope with withdrawal symptoms and cravings. Be aware that you should not chew nicotine gum as you would chew ordinary gum. Instead, first chew slowly until you can taste the peppery flavor of the nicotine, or until you feel a slight tingling sensation in your mouth. This generally requires about fifteen chews. Then stop chewing and park (place) the gum between your cheek and gums for about a minute—just until the taste or tingling sensation stops. Chew the gum as before, and park as before, being careful to park the gum in a different spot in your mouth each time to prevent irritation. Continue to alternately chew and park for about thirty minutes, at which point most of the nicotine will have been released from the gum. Discard the gum, and rinse your mouth with water or mouthwash. Remember that most of the time the gum is in your mouth, it should be parked.

Opinions vary regarding the frequency with which you should chew nicotine gum. Some say that you should use it on a regular basis—say, every one to two hours—to prevent withdrawal symptoms and cravings. Others recommend that you chew the gum only when you need it—for instance, when a craving hits or when withdrawal symptoms appear. Follow the manufacturer's directions regarding the frequency with which you chew the gum, as well as the number of pieces used each day. Generally, it is recommended that regardless of the strength of the gum, you chew about eight to twelve pieces each day, using no more than twenty-four pieces daily unless you are under the supervision of a doctor.

It is generally suggested that you start to reduce the amount of nicotine gum used after two months, and that you use it no longer than three months. To reduce the use of the gum, you can, over time, decrease the number of pieces used each day; decrease the chewing time used for each piece; substitute one or more pieces of regular sugarless gum for some of the nicotine gum; or substitute 2-milligram gum for 4-milligram gum. Be aware that if you stop using the gum abruptly, you may experience the same withdrawal symptoms caused by abrupt cessation of smoking. If you find it impossible to quit using the gum six months after beginning nicotine replacement therapy, be sure to continue gum use only under a doctor's supervision.

Although nicotine gum can help you quit smoking, it's important to understand that the gum alone will not enable you to give up cigarettes. Smokers are addicted not just to nicotine, but to the entire smoking experience. For that reason, you'll have greatest success using the gum if you anticipate possible problems and have some solutions on hand. Note, too, that because the gum delivers a drug into your system, you'll want to take certain precautions to make the quitting experience as safe as possible. These tips should help:

❑ As discussed in Part One (see page 28), you will more effectively use *any* method of quitting if before beginning, you identify your core values. For instance, your core value may be maintaining good health so that you can continue to participate in your favorite sports throughout your life. If you remember this core value and keep it foremost in your mind, it will be all the easier for you to keep away from cigarettes.

❑ If possible, get help from a stop-smoking program that includes either individual or group counseling. These programs—which provide encouragement and guide you in avoiding common mistakes—can double your chance of success. (See page 34 for more information.)

❑ Tell friends and family members that you have quit, and reach out to them for help when you need it. Some smokers use cigarettes as their support. If this is true of you, now is the time to make a change. I think you'll find that humans make a far better support group than a pack of cigarettes.

❑ Use of the nicotine gum should help satisfy the need to have something in your mouth in place of a cigarette. When you're not chewing the gum, try toothpicks, cinnamon sticks, lollipops or other hard candy, sugar-free gum, or carrot or celery sticks.

❑ If you miss holding a cigarette in your hand, replace it with a pencil, a paper clip, a marble, or a bottle of water.

❑ Keep your hands (and your mind) busy. Do crossword puzzles or needlework; try sketching or painting; clean closets; do woodworking or gardening.

❑ Try to avoid your usual triggers. If you always light up when taking a coffee break with your coworkers, skip your usual break routine and, instead, take a walk or catch up on your reading. If you enjoy a cigarette at the dinner table after your meal, get up from the table as soon as you finish eating. Cigarette smoking is a habit as well as an addiction, and habits can be broken.

❏ When a craving hits, you will sometimes be able to combat it by chewing a piece of nicotine gum. At other times, close your eyes and count slowly down from ten to zero, breathing deeply with each count. If that doesn't work, call a friend or take a walk—even if it's just to the end of your driveway. The trick is to find some diversion until the craving passes. And it will.

❏ If you're concerned about gaining weight as the result of quitting, keep healthy foods within easy reach. Those vegetable sticks will not only keep your hands busy but will also help you deal with the hunger that often results when the appetite-suppressant action of cigarettes is no longer at work. Also drink plenty of water and eat plenty of fresh fruit.

❏ Exercise. It will not only fight weight gain, but will also keep both your hands and your mind busy, providing a healthy distraction from any cravings. In fact, exercise can support your quit-smoking efforts in many ways. (To learn more, see "Exercise—A Powerful Tool Against Smoking" on page 44.)

❏ If the sight of other people smoking makes you want to reach for a cigarette, stop, and make a mental switch as discussed in Part One. (See page 36.) Instead of focusing on the great time the smokers appear to be having, think of how those cigarettes are flooding their bodies with toxins. Now picture your empty wallet, and remember what it's like to wake up with a smoker's cough. Finally, reconnect with your core values and use those values to strengthen your resolve.

❏ Don't be concerned if you find yourself coughing after you begin use of the gum. Although nicotine gum lessens the severity of withdrawal symptoms, you may still cough as your body rids itself of the tars and toxins that have accumulated through years of smoking. Accept this as a good sign— a sign of healing—and keep your throat as moist and comfortable as possible by drinking plenty of fluids and using throat lozenges.

❏ Resist the urge to have "just one more cigarette." Once you quit cold turkey, *you quit*. More important, using any NRT and smoking at the same time is dangerous because it can cause you to overdose on nicotine.

❏ Do not try to make quitting easier by using multiple forms of NRT, such as both the patch and nicotine gum, without medical supervision. This, too, can result in nicotine overdose. Use a combination of these tools only under the guidance of your doctor. (See "Can You Use More Than One NRT At a Time?" on page 75.)

❏ If you find yourself overwhelmed by cravings for nicotine, don't chew more than one piece of gum at a time, and don't chew a new piece too soon after finishing an old one. You should wait at least an hour between pieces. If the gum is not sufficiently controlling your cravings, speak to your doctor about combining the gum with a nicotine patch (see the inset on page 75), or about using other types of quit-smoking tools.

❏ Chew the nicotine gum *slowly* and for no more than the time specified by the manufacturer—usually, about thirty minutes. If the gum is chewed too quickly or for too long, you will produce a lot of saliva, which will carry some of the nicotine down your throat. You want the nicotine to be absorbed through your mouth, and not wasted through swallowing. Fast chewing can also lead to throat irritations, nausea, stomachache, hiccups, dizziness, and headaches.

❏ Avoiding eating and drinking—especially acidic beverages, such as coffee or soft drinks—for fifteen minutes before chewing the gum, or while you chew the gum. Drinking or eating too close to the time you use the gum will reduce absorption of the nicotine, making the gum less effective.

❏ Nicotine gum looks like candy to a child, so keep unused pieces away from children as well as from pets, and dispose of used gum where kids and pets can't get to it. It's important to remember that nicotine gum is a drug, and must be used with caution.

❏ Remember that the purpose of nicotine gum is to replace the nicotine your body is craving. Your body signals its craving with withdrawal symptoms. If you are not experiencing any withdrawal symptoms, or at least any significant withdrawal symptoms, you do not need to chew another piece of gum.

Keep in mind that even when using nicotine gum, quitting will require iron resolve. NRTs do not eliminate your emotional attachment to cigarettes, nor do they usually replace the full amount of nicotine you've been getting from cigarettes, so you may still have some mild withdrawal symptoms. Don't expect quitting to be a walk in the park just because you're using nicotine gum. But if you're determined to quit and you want to temper possible withdrawal symptoms, this gum may be the answer. It is easy to use, and has the advantage of helping you fight cravings when they occur.

HOW WELL DOES IT WORK?

Smoking is an addiction, and the addiction is different for every person. For that reason, the withdrawal process is more difficult for some smokers than it is for others even when nicotine gum is in use. But evidence shows that the gum can be effective. According to studies, 25 to 30 percent of people who use some form of nicotine replacement therapy are smoke-free six months after starting use of the NRT. After a year, NRTs appears to be about twice as effective as quitting cold turkey without any aids. Note that nicotine gum has been found to be neither more nor less effective than the nicotine patch and nicotine lozenges. The rate of success appears to be the same for these three forms of NRT.

RISKS AND DISADVANTAGES

To start, it's important to understand that using any nicotine replacement therapy, including gum, is much safer for you than smoking cigarettes. Remember that cigarettes contain thousands of toxic chemicals, while an NRT supplies only nicotine.

Can You Use More Than One NRT At a Time?

Some smokers feel that if one NRT is good, several are even better. So on their own—with the idea of preventing any and all withdrawal symptoms—they chew the gum, wear the patch, and maybe even suck on a nicotine lozenge now and then.

As mentioned on page 73, you should *not* combine several forms of NRT on your own, as this can lead to a dangerous overdose of nicotine. But if you feel that you need more help than the gum provides, by all means speak to your doctor about the judicious use of two types of nicotine replacement therapy. You may, for instance, use the patch to provide a continual low level of nicotine delivery, and then chew nicotine gum once in a while to deal with breakthrough withdrawal symptoms. As the weeks go by, you will taper down the use of both the gum and the patch, until you are free of nicotine.

Yes, the use of two types of NRT can help keep withdrawal symptoms at bay. Just be sure to get your doctor's okay, and to use these powerful quit-smoking tools exactly as your physician directs.

With that said, it's impossible to overemphasize the fact that nicotine gum is a drug, and that it must be used with caution. It's a good idea to discuss the gum with your doctor before purchasing it. He or she can guide you in choosing the best strength gum for your needs, and help monitor any problems throughout the quitting process. Moreover, if your physician prescribes the NRT, your health insurance may actually cover it, making it more affordable.

Most important, though, you must confer with your doctor if you are pregnant, planning to become pregnant, or nursing; if you are under the age of eighteen; or if you have one of the following conditions:

- Asthma
- Cardiovascular disease, including angina pectoris (chest pain), arrhythmia, and recent heart attack
- Diabetes
- High blood pressure
- Impaired circulation
- Kidney disease
- Liver disease
- Lung disease, such as emphysema
- Pheochromocytoma (a tumor of the adrenal gland)
- Recurrent nasal allergies
- Stomach ulcer
- Thyroid problems

One or more of the above conditions won't necessarily rule out use of nicotine gum. In the case of heart disease, for instance, although nicotine replacement therapy may not be the treatment of choice, your doctor may feel that the gum poses a far lesser risk than that of continued smoking. In some cases, though, your physician may recommend a product that's a better match for your individual risk profile.

When discussing the possible use of an NRT with your doctor, be sure to mention all the medications you're currently taking, including prescription drugs and over-the-counter medications. Especially tell your doctor if you are taking one of the following:

- Acetaminophen (Tylenol and others)

- Caffeine

- Diuretics (water pills)

- Imipramine (Tofranil, Janimine)

- Insulin

- High blood pressure medications

- Oxazepam (Serax)

- Pentazocine (Talwin, Talwin NX, Talacen)

- Propoxyphene (Darvon, Darvon-N, E-Lor, PC-CAP, Wygesic, and others)

- Propranolol (Inderal)

- Theophylline (Aerolate, Asmalix, Theo-Dur, and others)

- Vitamins

Again, use of any of the above substances may not rule out the use of nicotine gum. But in some cases, your doctor may suggest a different quit-smoking technique.

Like all NRTs, nicotine gum can cause side effects. The side effects most often associated with gum use include the following:

- Abdominal pain

- Blurred vision

- Diarrhea or upset stomach

- Dizziness

- Headaches

- Hiccups

- High blood pressure

- Jaw muscle aches

- Mouth ulcers

- Nausea and/or vomiting

- Weakness

Some side effects, like hiccups and sore jaw muscles, are usually due to improper chewing, and most occur only during the first few weeks. If these

The Pros and Cons of Nicotine Gum

The Pros

❏ It's available over-the-counter.

❏ It's easy to use.

❏ It lessens withdrawal symptoms and cravings by supplying nicotine.

❏ Because it delivers nicotine only when chewed, it can help mimic the highs and lows of cigarette smoking.

❏ Because it looks like candy, it can be used fairly inconspicuously.

❏ It satisfies the need to have something in your mouth.

❏ If you get a prescription from your doctor, it may be covered by your insurance.

The Cons

❏ It must be purchased.

❏ Because it's a drug, people with certain medical problems cannot use it.

❏ It must be used carefully, and can cause side effects.

❏ Because it is thick and sticky, it is not a good choice for people with temporomandibular joint disease (TMJ) or for people with braces, dentures, bridges, or major dental restoration.

symptoms persist, however, you should contact your physician to determine if it is safe for you to continue using the gum. Contact your physician *immediately* if you have any of the following problems, which may be signs of nicotine overdose.

- Abnormal heartbeat or rhythm
- Cold sweats
- Difficulty breathing
- Salivating
- Seizures
- Severe abdominal pain
- Tremors

The lists of potential side effects presented on earlier pages are not meant to scare you, but to make you aware of the possible consequences of nicotine use or overdose so that you will be alert to problems. Similarly, it's important to understand fully that *you should not smoke when using nicotine gum or any other NRT.* This can cause a serious nicotine overdose, which can result in death.

Finally, it should be noted that aside from being a drug, nicotine gum is a rather thick and sticky substance—more viscous than regular chewing gum. For that reason, people with temporomandibular joint disease (TMJ) should probably not use nicotine gum, as it may exacerbate the condition. Also, because the gum tends to adhere to dental work, it may be unsuitable for people with braces, dentures, bridges, or significant dental restoration.

CONCLUSION

Nicotine gum is a readily available over-the-counter aid that can help you quit smoking cold turkey by reducing or eliminating your withdrawal symptoms. Despite the gum's possible side effects, many people have already used this type of nicotine replacement therapy safely. In fact, less than 5 percent of the people who try nicotine gum have to stop use due to side effects. And as mentioned earlier, studies show that the gum can actually *double* your chance of successfully quitting the smoking habit.

Just keep in mind that like any aid, nicotine gum will be effective only if you pair it with motivation and willpower. No form of nicotine replacement therapy can quit smoking for you, but if you access your core values and cement your motivation before your Quit Date, the gum can certainly help you get through the quitting process.

Remember, too, that although nicotine gum is one of the best known quit-smoking aids, it is not the only aid. For that reason, before settling on the gum, you may want to consider some of the other options available. Perhaps you would have more success if you used another type of NRT, such as the patch or nicotine lozenges. Or perhaps you can maximize your success by using the gum along with another tool, such as hypnosis. In the following chapters, you'll learn about other quit-smoking aids that can help you as you move towards a smoke-free lifestyle.

#5

Nicotine Lozenges

Some quitting methods, like cold turkey and tapering, essentially rely on willpower to cope with withdrawal symptoms and cravings. But the fact is that the physical symptoms caused by nicotine withdrawal are one of the primary reasons that people return to smoking. Willpower isn't always enough.

Nicotine replacement therapy (NRT) was designed to reduce withdrawal symptoms by supplying a relatively safe source of nicotine in measured doses that can be reduced in strength or frequency until the supply of nicotine is completely stopped. This therapy has helped many people successfully stop smoking.

Several types of NRT are now on the market. Nicotine patches, gum, and lozenges are available without a prescription, while nicotine nasal sprays and inhalers are available through prescription only. This chapter will examine nicotine lozenges so that you can decide if they would help you in your efforts to quit smoking. See Chapters 3, 4, 6, and 7 to learn about the other forms of nicotine replacement therapy.

WHAT IS IT?

The nicotine lozenge is an oral form of nicotine therapy that is much like a hard candy, except that it contains nicotine. As the lozenge dissolves in the mouth, it slowly releases all of the nicotine, allowing it to be absorbed by the body.

Like nicotine gum, discussed in the previous chapter, the lozenge comes in different strengths—2 milligrams and 4 milligrams—so that smokers can use the strength that is appropriate for the amount of nicotine they are used to getting from cigarettes. (The average cigarette delivers roughly 2 milligrams of nicotine, with some containing less and some containing more.) Lozenges are available in different flavors, such as mint and cherry.

This type of NRT is intended to be used as needed, whenever the craving to smoke arises.

HOW DOES IT WORK?

As you learned earlier in the book, the nicotine in cigarettes provides feelings of enjoyment by increasing brain levels of the chemical dopamine—a substance associated with the pleasure system of the brain. As nicotine creates a feeling of pleasure time and time again, it also creates an addiction that causes your brain to punish you when smoking stops. When the supply of tobacco is severed, you experience symptoms such as irritability, frustration, anxiety, restlessness, and insomnia. Many people find these symptoms so distressing that they start smoking cigarettes again despite their desire to quit.

Nicotine lozenges help you stop smoking by bringing nicotine into your body via a different delivery system—a safer delivery system that does not provide the tars, carbon monoxide, and other toxic chemicals contained in cigarettes. As the lozenge dissolves in your mouth, the nicotine is released and absorbed through the mucous membranes of your mouth into your bloodstream. Because your brain is not starved of nicotine, it produces either no withdrawal symptoms or less severe symptoms, making it easier to quit.

It's important to understand that all NRTs work in different ways. The patch, discussed in Chapter 3, delivers a slow, constant, low level of nicotine. But like nicotine gum, the lozenge delivers a measured dose of nicotine only when you place it in your mouth. This not only helps simulate the highs and lows of nicotine normally experienced when smoking cigarettes, but also acts as a substitute oral activity.

HOW DO YOU USE IT?

Nicotine lozenges must be used in combination with cold turkey quitting. You cannot smoke while using the lozenges, as this can result in an overdose of nicotine. For that reason, your first step in using this technique is to choose a Quit Date, just as you would if you were quitting cold turkey without the help of an NRT.

Next, you must choose the right strength lozenge. It is a good idea to speak to your physician or pharmacist regarding the best strength to use. Generally, manufacturers recommend that if you tend to smoke your first cigarette within thirty minutes of waking up, you use the 4-milligram lozenge. If you smoke your first cigarette *more* than thirty minutes after awakening, the 2-milligram lozenge may be a more appropriate choice.

When your Quit Date arrives and you stop smoking, you can begin using the nicotine lozenge as needed—whenever the craving to smoke a cigarette arises. To achieve best results and avoid unpleasant side effects, place the nicotine lozenge in your mouth and allow it to dissolve slowly. This should take twenty to thirty minutes. As you suck on the lozenge, occasionally move it from one side of your mouth to the other. Minimize swallowing, and do not chew or swallow the lozenge, as this will not only decrease your absorption of the nicotine, but can also lead to problems such as heartburn.

To prevent nicotine withdrawal symptoms, manufacturers generally recommend that you use at least nine lozenges a day for the first six weeks, and that you use no more than twenty during each twenty-four hour period. In other words, during waking hours, you can have about one lozenge an hour. After the first six weeks, you should start reducing your use of the NRT by increasing the interval between lozenges. For instance, you might use one lozenge every one to two hours for the first six weeks; one every two to four hours from week seven to week nine; and one every four to eight hours during the last three weeks. Be aware that if you stop using the lozenges abruptly, rather than tapering off, you may experience the same withdrawal symptoms caused by the abrupt cessation of smoking. If you feel that you still need to use the lozenges after twelve weeks, speak to your doctor.

Although nicotine lozenges can help you quit smoking, it's important to understand that the lozenges alone will not enable you to give up cigarettes. Smokers are addicted not just to nicotine, but to the entire smoking experience. For that reason, you'll have greatest success using the lozenges if you anticipate possible problems and have some solutions on hand. Note, too, that because the lozenges deliver a drug into your system, you'll want to take certain precautions to make the quitting experience as safe as possible. These tips should help:

❏ As discussed in Part One (see page 28), you will more effectively use *any* method of quitting if before beginning, you identify your core values. For

instance, your core value may be maintaining good health so that you can continue to participate in your favorite sports throughout your life. If you remember this core value and keep it foremost in your mind, it will be all the easier for you to keep away from cigarettes.

❏ If possible, get help from a stop-smoking program that includes either individual or group counseling. These programs—which provide encouragement and guide you in avoiding common mistakes—can double your chance of success. (See page 34 for more information.)

❏ Tell friends and family members that you have quit, and reach out to them for help when you need it. Some smokers use cigarettes as their support. If this is true of you, now is the time to make a change. I think you'll find that humans make a far better support group than a pack of cigarettes.

❏ Use of the nicotine lozenge should help satisfy the need to have something in your mouth in place of a cigarette. When you're not sucking on a lozenge, try toothpicks, cinnamon sticks, lollipops or other hard candy, sugar-free gum, or carrot or celery sticks.

❏ If you miss holding a cigarette in your hand, replace it with a pencil, a paper clip, a marble, or a bottle of water.

❏ Keep your hands (and your mind) busy. Do crossword puzzles or needlework; try sketching or painting; clean closets; do woodworking or gardening.

❏ Try to avoid your usual triggers. If you always light up when taking a coffee break with your coworkers, skip your usual break routine and, instead, take a walk or catch up on your reading. If you enjoy a cigarette at the dinner table after your meal, get up from the table as soon as you finish eating. Cigarette smoking is a habit as well as an addiction, and habits can be broken.

❏ When a craving hits, you may be able to combat it by sucking on a nicotine lozenge. If it's not yet time for another lozenge, close your eyes and count slowly down from ten to zero, breathing deeply with each count. If that doesn't work, call a friend or take a walk—even if it's just to the end of your driveway. The trick is to find some diversion until the craving passes. And it will.

❏ If you're concerned about gaining weight as the result of quitting, keep healthy foods within easy reach. Those vegetable sticks will not only keep your hands busy but will also help you deal with the hunger that often results when the appetite-suppressant action of cigarettes is no longer at work. Also drink plenty of water and eat plenty of fresh fruit.

❏ Exercise. It will not only fight weight gain, but will also keep both your hands and your mind busy, providing a healthy distraction from any cravings. In fact, exercise can support your quit-smoking efforts in many ways. (To learn more, see "Exercise—A Powerful Tool Against Smoking" on page 44.)

❏ If the sight of other people smoking makes you want to reach for a cigarette, stop, and make a mental switch as discussed in Part One. (See page 36.) Instead of focusing on the great time the smokers appear to be having, think of how those cigarettes are flooding their bodies with toxins. Now picture your empty wallet, and remember what it's like to wake up with a smoker's cough. Finally, reconnect with your core values and use those values to strengthen your resolve.

❏ Don't be concerned if you find yourself coughing after you begin using the lozenges. Although use of an NRT lessens the severity of withdrawal symptoms, you may still cough as your body rids itself of the tars and toxins that have accumulated through years of smoking. Accept this as a good sign—a sign of healing—and keep your throat as moist and comfortable as possible by drinking plenty of fluids and using throat lozenges.

❏ Resist the urge to have "just one more cigarette." Once you quit cold turkey, *you quit.* More important, using any NRT and smoking at the same time is dangerous because it can cause you to overdose on nicotine.

❏ Do not try to make quitting easier by using multiple forms of NRT, such as both the lozenges and the patch, without medical supervision. This, too, can result in nicotine overdose. Use a combination of these tools only under the guidance of your doctor. (See "Can You Use More Than One NRT At a Time?" on page 87.)

❏ If you find yourself overwhelmed by cravings for nicotine, don't suck on more than one lozenge at a time, and don't use one after another, as this can cause hiccups, heartburn, nausea, and other side effects. Wait at least an hour between lozenges. If the lozenges are not sufficiently controlling your cravings, speak to your doctor about combining this NRT with other types of quit-smoking tools.

❏ Be sure to avoid chewing or swallowing the nicotine lozenge. If you chew it and swallow it as you might a hard candy, you will swallow the nicotine rather than absorbing it into your system to fight withdrawal symptoms. This will not only waste the nicotine, but can lead to hiccups, heartburn, nausea, and other unpleasant side effects.

❏ Avoid eating and drinking for fifteen minutes before using a lozenge, as well as while you're using a lozenge. Drinking or eating too close to the time you use this NRT will reduce absorption of the nicotine, making the lozenge less effective.

❏ Nicotine lozenges may look like candy to a child, so keep unused lozenges away from children as well as from pets, and if you choose to dispose of a lozenge after you start sucking on it, make sure that kids and pets can't get to it. It's important to remember that nicotine lozenges are a drug, and must be used with caution.

❏ Remember that the purpose of the nicotine lozenge is to replace the nicotine your body is craving. Your body signals its craving with withdrawal symptoms. If you are not experiencing any withdrawal symptoms, or at least any significant withdrawal symptoms, you do not need to suck on another lozenge.

Keep in mind that even when using nicotine lozenges, quitting will require iron resolve. NRTs do not eliminate your emotional attachment to cigarettes, nor do they usually replace the full amount of nicotine you've been getting from cigarettes, so you may still have some mild withdrawal symptoms. Don't expect quitting to be a walk in the park just because you're using nicotine lozenges. But if you're determined to quit and you want to temper possible withdrawal symptoms, this NRT may be the answer. It is easy to use; it can be used inconspicuously, without the obvious chewing necessary with nicotine gum; and it has the advantage of helping you fight cravings when they occur.

HOW WELL DOES IT WORK?

Smoking is an addiction, and the addiction is different for every person. For that reason, the withdrawal process is more difficult for some smokers than it is for others even when nicotine lozenges are used. But evidence shows that the lozenges can be effective. According to studies, 25 to 30 percent of people who use some form of nicotine replacement therapy are smoke-free six months after starting use of the NRT. After a year, NRTs appears to be about twice as effective as quitting cold turkey without any aids. Note that nicotine lozenges have been found to be neither more nor less effective than

Can You Use More Than One NRT At a Time?

Some smokers feel that if one NRT is good, several are even better. So on their own—with the idea of preventing any and all withdrawal symptoms—they suck on lozenges, wear the patch, and maybe even chew a piece of nicotine gum now and then.

As mentioned on page 85, you should *not* combine several forms of NRT on your own, as this can lead to a dangerous overdose of nicotine. But if you feel that you need more help than the lozenges provide, by all means speak to your doctor about the judicious use of two types of nicotine replacement therapy. You may, for instance, wear the patch to provide a continual low level of nicotine delivery, and use a nicotine lozenge once in a while to deal with breakthrough withdrawal symptoms. As the weeks go by, you will taper your use of both the lozenges and the patch, until you are free of nicotine.

Yes, the use of two types of NRT can help keep withdrawal symptoms at bay. Just be sure to get your doctor's okay, and to use these powerful quit-smoking tools exactly as your physician directs.

the nicotine patch and nicotine gum. The rate of success appears to be the same for these three forms of NRT.

RISKS AND DISADVANTAGES

To start, it's important to understand that using any nicotine replacement therapy, including lozenges, is much safer for you than smoking cigarettes. Remember that cigarettes contain thousands of toxic chemicals, while an NRT supplies only nicotine.

With that said, it's impossible to overemphasize the fact that the nicotine lozenge is a drug, and that it must be used with caution. It's a good idea to discuss the lozenges with your doctor before purchasing them. He or she can guide you in choosing the best strength product for your needs, and help monitor any problems throughout the quitting process. Moreover, if your physician prescribes the NRT, your health insurance may actually cover it, making it more affordable.

Most important, though, you must confer with your doctor if you are pregnant, planning to become pregnant, or nursing; if you are under the age of eighteen; or if you have one of the following conditions:

- Asthma

- Cardiovascular disease, including angina pectoris (chest pain), arrhythmia, and recent heart attack

- Diabetes

- High blood pressure

- Impaired circulation

- Kidney disease

- Liver disease

- Lung disease, such as emphysema

- Phenylketonuria

- Pheochromocytoma (a tumor of the adrenal gland)

- Recurrent nasal allergies

- Stomach ulcer

- Thyroid problems

One or more of the above conditions won't necessarily rule out use of nicotine lozenges. In the case of heart disease, for instance, although nicotine replacement therapy may not be the treatment of choice, your doctor may feel that the lozenges pose a lesser risk than that of continued smoking. In some cases, though, your physician may recommend a product that's a better match for your individual risk profile. People with phenylketonuria should be aware that many nicotine lozenges contain more than 3 milligrams of phenylalanine each. This substance is not found in other forms of NRT.

When discussing the possible use of an NRT with your doctor, be sure to mention all the medications you're currently taking, including prescription drugs and over-the-counter medications. Especially tell your doctor if you are taking one of the following:

- Acetaminophen (Tylenol and others)

- Caffeine

- Diuretics (water pills)

- Imipramine (Tofranil, Janimine)

- Insulin

- High blood pressure medications

- Oxazepam (Serax)

- Pentazocine (Talwin, Talwin NX, Talacen)

- Propoxyphene (Darvon, Darvon-N, E-Lor, PC-CAP, Wygesic, and others)

- Propranolol (Inderal)

- Theophylline (Aerolate, Asmalix, Theo-Dur, and others)

- Vitamins

Again, use of any of the above substances may not rule out the use of nicotine lozenges. But in some cases, your doctor may suggest a different quit-smoking technique.

Like all NRTs, nicotine lozenges can cause side effects. The side effects most often associated with lozenge use include the following:

- Abdominal pain

- Blurred vision

- Diarrhea or upset stomach

- Dizziness

- Excess gas (flatulence)

- Headaches

- Heartburn

- Hiccups

- High blood pressure

- Nausea and/or vomiting

- Sore throat

- Weakness

Some side effects, like heartburn and indigestion, are usually due to improper use of the nicotine lozenge. Practices such as chewing the lozenges, swallowing the lozenges whole, or using them one after another can all cause problems. When the lozenges are used properly, most symptoms occur only during the first few weeks. If symptoms persist, however, you should contact your physician to determine if it is safe for you to continue using the lozenges. Contact your physician *immediately* if you have any of the following problems, which may be signs of nicotine overdose.

- Abnormal heartbeat or rhythm

- Cold sweats

- Difficulty breathing

- Seizures

- Severe abdominal pain

- Tremors

The Pros and Cons of the Nicotine Lozenge

The Pros

❏ It's available over-the-counter.

❏ It lessens withdrawal symptoms and cravings by supplying nicotine.

❏ Because it delivers nicotine only when used, it can help mimic the highs and lows of cigarette smoking.

❏ It's easy to use.

❏ Because it looks like candy, it can be used inconspicuously.

❏ It satisfies the need to have something in your mouth.

❏ If you get a prescription from your doctor, it may be covered by your insurance.

The Cons

❏ It must be purchased.

❏ Because it's a drug, people with certain medical problems cannot use it.

❏ It must be used carefully, and can cause side effects.

❏ Because it is sticky, it can adhere to dental work, and might not be a good choice for people with braces, dentures, bridges, or major dental restoration.

The lists of potential side effects presented on previous pages are not meant to scare you, but to make you aware of the possible consequences of nicotine use or overdose so that you will be alert to problems. Similarly, it's important to understand fully that *you should not smoke when using nicotine lozenges or any other NRT.* This can cause a serious nicotine overdose, which can result in death.

Finally, it should be noted that aside from being a drug, nicotine lozenges are sticky and can adhere to dental work. For that reason, they may be unsuitable for people with braces, dentures, bridges, or significant dental restoration.

CONCLUSION

The nicotine lozenge is a readily available over-the-counter aid that can help you quit smoking cold turkey by reducing or eliminating your withdrawal symptoms. Despite the lozenge's possible side effects, many people have already used this type of nicotine replacement therapy safely. In fact, less than 5 percent of the people who try nicotine lozenges have to stop use due to side effects. And as mentioned earlier, studies show that the lozenges can actually *double* your chance of successfully quitting the smoking habit.

Just keep in mind that like any aid, nicotine lozenges will be effective only if you pair them with motivation and willpower. No form of nicotine replacement therapy can quit smoking for you, but if you access your core values and cement your motivation before your Quit Date, the lozenges can certainly help you get through the quitting process.

Remember, too, that these lozenges are not the only quit-smoking aid available. For that reason, before settling on an aid, you may want to consider some of the other options available. Perhaps you would have more success if you used another type of NRT, such as the patch. Or perhaps you can maximize your success by using the lozenges along with another tool, such as hypnosis. The other chapters in Part Two are packed with information about additional quit-smoking aids that can help you as you move towards a smoke-free lifestyle.

#6

Nicotine Nasal Spray

Some quitting methods, like cold turkey and tapering, essentially rely on willpower to cope with withdrawal symptoms and cravings. But the fact is that the physical symptoms caused by nicotine withdrawal are one of the primary reasons that people return to smoking. Willpower isn't always enough.

Nicotine replacement therapy (NRT) was designed to reduce withdrawal symptoms by supplying a relatively safe source of nicotine in measured doses that can be reduced in strength or frequency until the supply of nicotine is completely stopped. This therapy has helped many people successfully stop smoking.

Several types of NRT are now on the market. Nicotine patches, gum, and lozenges are available without a prescription, while nicotine nasal sprays and inhalers are available through prescription only. This chapter will examine the nicotine nasal spray so that you can decide if it would help you in your efforts to quit smoking. See Chapters 3, 4, 5, and 7 to learn about the other forms of nicotine replacement therapy.

WHAT IS IT?

The nicotine nasal spray dispenses small doses of nicotine into the nasal passages, where it can be absorbed by the body. Each spray bottle contains 100 milligrams of nicotine in a concentration of 10 milligrams per milliliter. Each individual spray delivers approximately 0.5 milligram of nicotine, with each bottle containing about 200 applications. Generally, a dose is considered two sprays, one in each nostril, which together deliver about 1 milligram of nicotine—about half the amount you would get by smoking a cigarette.

This type of NRT is intended to be used on a regular basis as a means of preventing or minimizing withdrawal symptoms.

HOW DOES IT WORK?

As you learned earlier in the book, the nicotine in cigarettes provides feelings of enjoyment by increasing brain levels of the chemical dopamine—a substance associated with the pleasure system of the brain. As nicotine creates a feeling of pleasure time and time again, it also creates an addiction that causes your brain to punish you when smoking stops. When the supply of tobacco is severed, you experience symptoms such as irritability, frustration, anxiety, restlessness, and insomnia. Many people find these symptoms so distressing that they start smoking cigarettes again despite their desire to quit.

Nicotine nasal spray helps you stop smoking by bringing nicotine into your body via a different delivery system—a safer delivery system that does not provide the tars, carbon monoxide, and other toxic chemicals contained in cigarettes. When the spray enters your nasal passages, it is absorbed into your bloodstream through the mucous membranes. Because your brain is not starved of nicotine, it produces either no withdrawal symptoms or less severe symptoms, making it easier to quit.

It's important to understand that all NRTs work in different ways. The patch delivers a slow, constant, low level of nicotine. But like nicotine gum and lozenges, the nasal spray delivers a measured dose of nicotine only when you choose to use it.

HOW DO YOU USE IT?

Nicotine nasal spray must be used in combination with cold turkey quitting. You cannot smoke while using the spray, as this can result in an overdose of nicotine. For that reason, your first step in using this technique is to choose a Quit Date, just as you would if you were quitting cold turkey without the help of an NRT.

Because nicotine nasal spray is not an over-the-counter product, you must discuss this quit-smoking tool with your doctor and—if the spray appears to be a safe option for you—obtain a prescription. Depending on your health insurance, this NRT may or may not be covered.

When your Quit Date arrives and you stop smoking, you should begin using your nicotine nasal spray according to the manufacturer's directions and your physician's recommendations. To use, simply prime the pump of the bottle, tilt your head back slightly, insert the tip of the bottle into one nostril, and spray once. For a complete dose, this should be repeated in the other nostril. (One dose consists of two sprays.) During this process, you must be careful to breathe through your mouth and to avoid sniffing or inhaling. You want the spray to remain in your nasal passages so that it can be absorbed through the mucous membranes. Be sure to avoid contact between the spray and your skin, mouth, eyes, and ears. If even a small amount of spray comes in contact with any of these areas of the body, immediately rinse the area with water only.

Along with your doctor, decide the frequency with which you will use the spray each day. The manufacturer suggests that you start with one or two doses each hour, with each dose consisting of two sprays, one in each nostril. This can be increased up to the maximum recommended dose of forty doses, or about half the bottle, per day. To prevent nicotine withdrawal symptoms, it is suggested that you use a minimum of eight doses per day, as fewer doses than this are likely to be ineffective. In clinical trials, it was found that people were most successful at quitting when they used the product more heavily during the peak of nicotine withdrawal.

You and your doctor should discuss the duration of your treatment and a method for eventually discontinuing use of the spray. You can, for example, use your agreed-upon number of daily doses for about eight weeks, and then taper the doses for four to six weeks before completely ending use. The maximum recommended duration of treatment is three months. Possible strategies for discontinuing use include using only a half dose (one spray) at a time, using the spray less frequently, skipping every other dose, or simply setting a planned Quit Date for ending use of the NRT. At this point, no method of tapering has been clinically proven to be superior to another.

Although nicotine nasal spray can help you quit smoking, it's important to understand that the spray alone will not enable you to give up cigarettes. Smokers are addicted not just to nicotine, but to the entire smoking experience. For that reason, you'll have greatest success using the spray if you anticipate possible problems and have some solutions on hand. Note, too, that because the spray contains a powerful drug, you'll want to take certain precautions to make the quitting experience as safe as possible. These tips should help:

❏ As discussed in Part One (see page 28), you will more effectively use *any* method of quitting if before beginning, you identify your core values. For

instance, your core value may be maintaining good health so that you can continue to participate in your favorite sports throughout your life. If you remember this core value and keep it foremost in your mind, it will be all the easier for you to keep away from cigarettes.

❑ If possible, get help from a stop-smoking program that includes either individual or group counseling. These programs—which provide encouragement and guide you in avoiding common mistakes—can double your chance of success. (See page 34 for more information.)

❑ Tell friends and family members that you have quit, and reach out to them for help when you need it. Some smokers use cigarettes as their support. If this is true of you, now is the time to make a change. I think you'll find that humans make a far better support group than a pack of cigarettes.

❑ If you miss having a cigarette in your mouth, try toothpicks, cinnamon sticks, lollipops or other hard candy, sugar-free gum, or carrot or celery sticks.

❑ If you miss holding a cigarette in your hand, replace it with a pencil, a paper clip, a marble, or a bottle of water.

❑ Keep your hands (and your mind) busy. Do crossword puzzles or needlework; try sketching or painting; clean closets; do woodworking or gardening.

❑ Try to avoid your usual triggers. If you always light up when taking a coffee break with your coworkers, skip your usual break routine and, instead, take a walk or catch up on your reading. If you enjoy a cigarette at the dinner table after your meal, get up from the table as soon as you finish eating. Cigarette smoking is a habit as well as an addiction, and habits can be broken.

❑ When a craving hits, you may be able to combat it by using the nicotine nasal spray. If it's not yet time for another dose, close your eyes and count slowly down from ten to zero, breathing deeply with each count. If that doesn't work, call a friend or take a walk—even if it's just to the end of your driveway. The trick is to find some diversion until the tobacco craving passes. And it will.

❑ If you're concerned about gaining weight as the result of quitting, keep healthy foods within easy reach. Those vegetable sticks will not only keep your hands busy but will also help you deal with the hunger that often results when the appetite-suppressant action of cigarettes is no longer at work. Also drink plenty of water and eat plenty of fresh fruit.

❑ Exercise. It will not only fight weight gain, but will also keep both your hands and your mind busy, providing a healthy distraction from any cravings for tobacco. In fact, exercise can support your quit-smoking efforts in many ways. (To learn more, see "Exercise—A Powerful Tool Against Smoking" on page 44.)

❑ If the sight of other people smoking makes you want to reach for a cigarette, stop, and make a mental switch as discussed in Part One. (See page 36.) Instead of focusing on the great time the smokers appear to be having, think of how those cigarettes are flooding their bodies with toxins. Now picture your empty wallet, and remember what it's like to wake up with a smoker's cough. Finally, reconnect with your core values and use those values to strengthen your resolve.

❑ Resist the urge to have "just one more cigarette." Once you quit cold turkey, *you quit.* More important, using any NRT and smoking at the same time is dangerous because it can cause you to overdose on nicotine.

❑ Do not try to make quitting easier by using multiple forms of NRT, such as the nasal spray and the patch, without medical supervision. This, too, can result in nicotine overdose. Use a combination of these tools only under the guidance of your doctor. (See "Can You Use More Than One NRT At a Time?" on page 98.)

❑ Don't be overly concerned if, when you first begin using the spray, you experience nose and throat irritations, coughing, sneezing, runny nose, and watery eyes. These are very common problems during the first week of treatment, but usually go away by the second week. If the symptoms don't disappear, or if you have any doubts about the seriousness of what you're experiencing, contact your doctor. (See page 100 for more about potential side effects.)

❑ Children and pets can be seriously harmed by even a small amount of nicotine, so be sure to keep the nasal spray away from them.

Keep in mind that even when using the nicotine nasal spray, quitting will require iron resolve. NRTs do not eliminate your emotional attachment to cigarettes, nor do they usually replace the full amount of nicotine you've been getting from cigarettes, so you may still have some mild withdrawal symptoms. Don't expect quitting to be a walk in the park just because you're using the spray. But if you're determined to quit and you want to temper possible withdrawal symptoms, this NRT may be the answer.

Can You Use More Than One NRT At a Time?

Some smokers feel that if one NRT is good, several are even better. So on their own—with the idea of preventing any and all withdrawal symptoms—they use the patch as well as their prescription nicotine nasal spray.

As mentioned on page 97, you should *not* combine several forms of NRT on your own, as this can lead to a dangerous overdose of nicotine. But if you feel that you need more help than the spray provides, by all means speak to your doctor about the judicious use of the patch along with the spray. Studies have shown that this combination of treatments can be more successful than the use of one NRT alone. Just be sure to use these powerful quit-smoking tools exactly as your physician directs.

HOW WELL DOES IT WORK?

Smoking is an addiction, and the addiction is different for every person. For that reason, the withdrawal process is more difficult for some smokers than it is for others even when the nicotine spray is used. But evidence shows that the spray can be effective. According to studies, 25 to 30 percent of people who use some form of nicotine replacement therapy are smoke-free six months after starting use of the NRT. After a year, NRTs appears to be about twice as effective as quitting cold turkey without any aids.

RISKS AND DISADVANTAGES

To start, it's important to understand that using any nicotine replacement therapy, including the nasal spray, is much safer than smoking cigarettes. Remember that cigarettes contain thousands of toxic chemicals, while an NRT supplies only nicotine.

With that said, it's impossible to overemphasize the fact that the nicotine nasal spray is a prescription drug, and that it must be used exactly as your doctor recommends. He or she will guide you in determining the frequency with which you use the spray, and the manner in which you decrease and stop use of the product. Since it is a prescription drug, your health insurance may cover it, making it more affordable.

Most important, though, you must tell your doctor if you are pregnant, planning to become pregnant, or nursing; if you are under the age of eighteen; or if you have one of the following conditions:

- Asthma

- Cardiovascular disease, including angina pectoris (chest pain), arrhythmia, and recent heart attack

- Chronic nasal disorders, including allergies, rhinitis, nasal polyps, and sinusitis

- Diabetes

- High blood pressure

- Impaired circulation

- Kidney disease

- Liver disease

- Lung disease, such as emphysema

- Pheochromocytoma (a tumor of the adrenal gland)

- Reactive airway disease

- Stomach ulcer

- Thyroid problems

One or more of the above conditions won't necessarily rule out use of nicotine nasal spray. In the case of heart disease, for instance, although nicotine replacement therapy may not be the treatment of choice, your doctor may feel that the spray poses a lesser risk than that of continued smoking. In some cases, though, your physician may recommend a product that's a better match for your individual risk profile. Because nicotine nasal spray is irritating to the breathing passages, it is generally not a good choice for people with breathing problems such as asthma, allergies, and sinus conditions. Another NRT, such as the patch or nicotine gum, would probably be a better quit-smoking tool in such a case.

When discussing the possible use of an NRT with your doctor, be sure to mention all the medications you're currently taking, including prescription drugs and over-the-counter medications. Especially tell your doctor if you are using one of the following:

- Acetaminophen (Tylenol and others)

- Beta-blockers, such as propranolol (Inderal)

- Caffeine

- Diuretics (water pills)
- Imipramine (Tofranil, Janimine)
- Insulin
- High blood pressure medications
- Nasal decongestants
- Oxazepam (Serax)
- Pentazocine (Talwin, Talwin NX, Talacen)
- Propoxyphene (Darvon, Darvon-N, E-Lor, PC-CAP, Wygesic, and others)
- Theophylline (Aerolate, Asmalix, Theo-Dur, and others)
- Vitamins

Again, use of any of the above substances may not rule out the use of nicotine nasal spray. But in some cases, your doctor may suggest a different quit-smoking technique.

Like all NRTs, nicotine nasal sprays can cause side effects. These side effects can include the following:

- Abdominal pain
- Blurred vision
- Coughing
- Diarrhea or upset stomach
- Dizziness
- Headaches
- High blood pressure
- Hot, peppery feeling in back of throat
- Nausea and/or vomiting
- Runny nose
- Shortness of breath
- Sore throat
- Sneezing
- Watery eyes
- Weakness

Some side effects, like high blood pressure, can occur with any NRT, because they are due to the action of the nicotine. Others—a burning feeling in the throat, coughing, runny nose, sneezing, and watery eyes—are very common in the first week or so of nasal spray use. However, if use is continued, the spray-specific symptoms usually go away. If these symptoms continue beyond the first week or so, or if you experience symptoms such as shortness of breath, contact your physician to determine if it is safe for you to continue using the spray. Contact your physician *immediately* if you have any of the following problems, which may be signs of nicotine overdose.

- Abnormal heartbeat or rhythm
- Difficulty breathing
- Seizures
- Severe abdominal pain

The Pros and Cons of Nicotine Nasal Spray

The Pros

❏ It lessens withdrawal symptoms and cravings by supplying nicotine.

❏ Because it delivers nicotine only when used, it can help mimic the highs and lows of cigarette smoking.

❏ It may be covered by your insurance.

The Cons

❏ You need a prescription to get it.

❏ Because it's a drug, people with certain medical problems cannot use it.

❏ It must be used carefully, and can cause side effects.

❏ Because of initial side effects, some people give up using it during the first week.

❏ It's conspicuous.

❏ It doesn't satisfy the need to have something in your mouth.

The lists of potential side effects presented on previous pages are not meant to scare you, but to make you aware of the possible consequences of nicotine use or overdose so that you will be alert to problems. Similarly, it's important to understand fully that *you should not smoke when using the nicotine nasal spray or any other NRT.* This can cause a serious nicotine overdose, which can result in death.

In addition to being aware of the potential risks and side effects of the nasal spray, it makes sense to understand its drawbacks. First, as you already know, you need a prescription to get the spray, making it less readily available than, say, nicotine gum. Second, it is not totally inconspicuous like the patch, nor can it masquerade as candy or cough drops like nicotine gum and lozenges. This high visibility bothers some people. Finally, unlike nicotine gum, nicotine lozenges, and the nicotine inhaler, the spray does not give you anything to put in your mouth.

CONCLUSION

Available by prescription, the nicotine nasal spray can help you quit smoking cold turkey by reducing or eliminating your withdrawal symptoms. Despite the spray's possible side effects, many people have already used this type of nicotine replacement therapy safely. And as mentioned earlier, studies show that the spray can actually *double* your chance of successfully quitting the smoking habit.

Just keep in mind that like any aid, the spray will be effective only if you pair it with motivation and willpower. No form of nicotine replacement therapy can quit smoking for you, but if you access your core values and cement your motivation before your Quit Date, the spray can certainly help you get through the quitting process.

Remember, too, that this spray is not the only quit-smoking aid available. For that reason, before settling on an aid, you may want to consider some of the other options available. Perhaps you would have more success if you used another type of NRT, such as the patch. Or perhaps you can maximize your success by using the spray along with another tool, such as hypnosis. The other chapters in Part Two are packed with information about additional quit-smoking aids that can help you as you move towards a smoke-free lifestyle.

#7

Nicotine Inhaler

Some quitting methods, like cold turkey and tapering, essentially rely on willpower to cope with withdrawal symptoms and cravings. But the fact is that the physical symptoms caused by nicotine withdrawal are one of the primary reasons that people return to smoking. Willpower isn't always enough.

Nicotine replacement therapy (NRT) was designed to lessen withdrawal symptoms by supplying a relatively safe source of nicotine in measured doses that can be reduced in strength or frequency until the supply of nicotine is completely stopped. This therapy has helped many people successfully stop smoking.

Several types of NRT are now on the market. Nicotine patches, gum, and lozenges are available without a prescription, while nicotine nasal sprays and inhalers are available through prescription only. This chapter will examine the nicotine inhaler so that you can decide if it would help you in your efforts to quit smoking. See Chapters 3, 4, 5, and 6 to learn about the other forms of nicotine replacement therapy.

WHAT IS IT?

The nicotine inhaler is a thin plastic device, the approximate shape and size of a cigarette, that holds a cartridge containing both nicotine and menthol. Each replaceable cartridge delivers about 80 puffs, or 2 milligrams of nicotine. (Although each cartridge contains 4 milligrams of nicotine, the body absorbs only 2 milligrams—roughly the amount provided by the average cigarette.) A single inhaler package contains one mouthpiece and a number of replaceable cartridges.

This NRT is intended to be used as needed to satisfy the craving for cigarettes and to prevent or minimize withdrawal symptoms.

HOW DOES IT WORK?

As you learned earlier in the book, the nicotine in cigarettes provides feelings of enjoyment by increasing brain levels of the chemical dopamine—a substance associated with the pleasure system of the brain. As nicotine creates a feeling of pleasure time and time again, it also creates an addiction that causes your brain to punish you when smoking stops. When the supply of tobacco is severed, you experience symptoms such as irritability, frustration, anxiety, restlessness, and insomnia. Many people find these symptoms so distressing that they start smoking cigarettes again despite their desire to quit.

The nicotine inhaler helps you stop smoking by bringing nicotine into your body via a different delivery system—a safer delivery system that does not provide the tars, carbon monoxide, and other toxic chemicals contained in cigarettes. When you puff on the inhaler, as you would puff on a cigarette, you extract a nicotine vapor that enters your mouth and throat, where it is absorbed into your bloodstream through the mucous membranes. Because your brain is not starved of nicotine, it produces either no withdrawal symptoms or less severe symptoms, making it easier to quit.

It's important to understand that all NRTs work in different ways. The patch, for instance, delivers a slow, constant, low level of nicotine. But the inhaler delivers nicotine only when you puff on it. This not only helps simulate the highs and lows of nicotine normally experienced when smoking cigarettes, but, through a familiar hand-to-mouth ritual, acts as a replacement for cigarettes.

HOW DO YOU USE IT?

The nicotine inhaler must be used in combination with cold turkey quitting. You cannot smoke while using the inhaler, as this can result in an overdose of nicotine. For that reason, your first step in using this technique is to choose a Quit Date, just as you would if you were quitting cold turkey without the help of an NRT.

Because the inhaler is not an over-the-counter product, you must discuss this quit-smoking tool with your doctor and—if the inhaler appears to be a safe option for you—obtain a prescription. Depending on your health insurance, this NRT may or may not be covered.

When your Quit Date arrives and you stop smoking, you should begin using your nicotine inhaler according to the manufacturer's directions and your physician's recommendations. Simply place the inhaler in your mouth and either inhale deeply into the back of your throat and mouth, or puff in short breaths. The nicotine will be used up after about twenty minutes of active puffing, or about eighty puffs. The best effects are achieved through frequent, continuous puffing.

Along with your doctor, decide the number of inhaler cartridges you will use each day. The manufacturer suggests that in the first three to twelve weeks, you use six to sixteen cartridges a day, as this will best help you through the nicotine withdrawal process. (Studies show that most people use about six cartridges a day.) Each day, you can try a different schedule to see what best meets your needs. For instance, you might want to use the inhaler for five minutes at a time, which would give you about four uses per cartridge. Or you might use the inhaler for ten-minute intervals. Be aware that when using the inhaler, less nicotine is released per puff than you would get from a cigarette. In addition, smokers report that puffs require more physical effort with an inhaler than with a cigarette. In other words, you must draw harder when using the inhaler.

You and your doctor should discuss the duration of your treatment and a method for eventually discontinuing use of the inhaler. You can, for example, use your agreed-upon number of daily cartridges for the first three to twelve weeks, and then gradually cut back on use. At this point, no method of tapering has been clinically proven to be superior to another, and some people have even found that they can stop abruptly with success. The maximum recommended duration of treatment is six months.

Although the nicotine inhaler can help you quit smoking, it's important to understand that the inhaler alone will not enable you to give up cigarettes. Smokers are addicted not just to nicotine, but to the entire smoking experience. For that reason, you'll have greatest success using this NRT if you anticipate possible problems and have some solutions on hand. Note, too, that because the inhaler delivers a powerful drug, you'll want to take certain precautions to make the quitting experience as safe as possible. These tips should help:

❑ As discussed in Part One (see page 28), you will more effectively use *any* method of quitting if before beginning, you identify your core values. For

instance, your core value may be maintaining good health so that you can continue to participate in your favorite sports throughout your life. If you remember this core value and keep it foremost in your mind, it will be all the easier for you to keep away from cigarettes.

❏ If possible, get help from a stop-smoking program that includes either individual or group counseling. These programs—which provide encouragement and guide you in avoiding common mistakes—can double your chance of success. (See page 34 for more information.)

❏ Tell friends and family members that you have quit, and reach out to them for help when you need it. Some smokers use cigarettes as their support. If this is true of you, now is the time to make a change. I think you'll find that humans make a far better support group than a pack of cigarettes.

❏ If you miss having a cigarette in your mouth, the inhaler should help, as it is puffed on much like a cigarette. When not using the inhaler, try toothpicks, cinnamon sticks, lollipops or other hard candy, sugar-free gum, or carrot or celery sticks.

❏ If you miss holding a cigarette in your hand, again, the inhaler should be a helpful cigarette replacement. When you start cutting down use, though, try holding a pencil, a paper clip, a marble, or a bottle of water.

❏ Keep your hands (and your mind) busy. Do crossword puzzles or needlework; try sketching or painting; clean closets; do woodworking or gardening.

❏ Try to avoid your usual triggers. If you always light up when taking a coffee break with your coworkers, skip your usual break routine and, instead, take a walk or catch up on your reading. If you enjoy a cigarette at the dinner table after your meal, get up from the table as soon as you finish eating. Cigarette smoking is a habit as well as an addiction, and habits can be broken.

❏ When a craving hits, you may be able to combat it by using your nicotine inhaler. If it's not yet time for another "dose," close your eyes and count slowly down from ten to zero, breathing deeply with each count. If that doesn't work, call a friend or take a walk—even if it's just to the end of your driveway. The trick is to find some diversion until the craving passes. And it will.

❏ If you're concerned about gaining weight as the result of quitting, keep healthy foods within easy reach. Those vegetable sticks will not only keep your hands busy but will also help you deal with the hunger that often results when the appetite-suppressant action of cigarettes is no longer at work. Also drink plenty of water and eat plenty of fresh fruit.

❏ Exercise. It will not only fight weight gain, but will also keep both your hands and your mind busy, providing a healthy distraction from any cravings. In fact, exercise can support your quit-smoking efforts in many ways. (To learn more, see "Exercise—A Powerful Tool Against Smoking" on page 44.)

❏ If the sight of other people smoking makes you want to reach for a cigarette, stop, and make a mental switch as discussed in Part One. (See page 36.) Instead of focusing on the great time the smokers appear to be having, think of how those cigarettes are flooding their bodies with toxins. Now picture your empty wallet, and remember what it's like to wake up with a smoker's cough. Finally, reconnect with your core values and use those values to strengthen your resolve.

❏ Resist the urge to have "just one more cigarette." Once you quit cold turkey, *you quit.* More important, using any NRT and smoking at the same time is dangerous because it can cause you to overdose on nicotine.

❏ Do not try to make quitting easier by using multiple forms of NRT, such as the inhaler and the patch, without medical supervision. This, too, can result in nicotine overdose. Use a combination of these tools *only* under the guidance of your doctor.

❏ Don't be overly concerned if, when you first begin using the inhaler, you experience irritation of your mouth and throat, a cough, a stuffy or runny nose, or an stomach upset. These are very common problems at the start of inhaler use, but usually go away in a short time if treatment is continued. If the symptoms don't disappear, or if you have any doubts about the seriousness of what you're experiencing, contact your doctor. (See page 110 for more about potential side effects.)

❏ Children and pets can be harmed by nicotine. Because even a used nicotine inhaler cartridge contains enough nicotine to cause a serious problem, it's vital to keep the inhaler away from children and pets.

Keep in mind that even when using the nicotine inhaler, quitting will require iron resolve. NRTs do not eliminate your emotional attachment to cigarettes, nor do they usually replace the full amount of nicotine you've been getting from cigarettes, so you may still have some mild withdrawal symptoms. Don't expect quitting to be a walk in the park just because you're using an NRT. But if you're determined to quit and you want to temper possible withdrawal symptoms with an aid that also acts as a cigarette substitute, the nicotine inhaler may be the answer.

HOW WELL DOES IT WORK?

Smoking is an addiction, and the addiction is different for every person. For that reason, the withdrawal process is more difficult for some smokers than it is for others even when the nicotine inhaler is used. But evidence shows that the inhaler can be effective. According to studies, 25 to 30 percent of people who use some form of nicotine replacement therapy are smoke-free six months after starting use of the NRT. After a year, NRTs appears to be about twice as effective as quitting cold turkey without any aids. And while no type of NRT has been proven more effective than another, some people prefer the inhaler because the process of handling the cartridge and puffing on it mimics the practice of smoking, making the inhaler a good cigarette substitute.

RISKS AND DISADVANTAGES

To start, it's important to understand that using any nicotine replacement therapy, including the inhaler, is much safer than smoking cigarettes. Remember that cigarettes contain thousands of toxic chemicals, while the inhaler supplies only nicotine and menthol.

With that said, it's impossible to overemphasize the fact that the nicotine inhaler is a prescription drug, and that it must be used exactly as your doctor recommends. He or she will guide you in determining the frequency with which you use the inhaler, and the manner in which you decrease and stop use of the product. Since it is a prescription drug, your health insurance may cover it, making it more affordable.

Most important, though, you must tell your doctor if you are pregnant, planning to become pregnant, or nursing; if you are under the age of eighteen; or if you have one of the following conditions:

- Asthma
- Cardiovascular disease, including angina pectoris (chest pain), arrhythmia, and recent heart attack
- Diabetes
- High blood pressure

- Impaired circulation

- Kidney disease

- Liver disease

- Lung disease, such as emphysema

- Pheochromocytoma (a tumor of the adrenal gland)

- Stomach ulcer

- Thyroid problems

One or more of the above conditions won't necessarily rule out use of nicotine nasal inhaler. In the case of heart disease, for instance, although nicotine replacement therapy may not be the treatment of choice, your doctor may feel that the inhaler poses a lesser risk than that of continued smoking. In some cases, though, your physician may recommend a product that's a better match for your individual risk profile.

When discussing the possible use of an NRT with your doctor, be sure to mention all the medications you're currently taking, including prescription drugs and over-the-counter medications. Especially tell your doctor if you are using one of the following:

- Acetaminophen (Tylenol and others)

- Beta-blockers, such as propranolol (Inderal)

- Caffeine

- Diuretics (water pills)

- Imipramine (Tofranil, Janimine)

- Insulin

- High blood pressure medications

- Nasal decongestants

- Oxazepam (Serax)

- Pentazocine (Talwin, Talwin NX, Talacen)

- Propoxyphene (Darvon, Darvon-N, E-Lor, PC-CAP, Wygesic, and others)

- Theophylline (Aerolate, Asmalix, Theo-Dur, and others)

- Vitamins

Again, use of any of the above substances may not rule out use of the nicotine inhaler. But in some cases, your doctor may suggest a different quit-smoking technique.

Like all NRTs, the nicotine inhaler can cause side effects. These side effects can include the following:

- Abdominal pain

- Blurred vision

- Coughing

- Diarrhea or upset stomach

- Dizziness

- Headaches

- High blood pressure

- Mouth irritation

- Nausea and/or vomiting

- Runny or stuffy nose

- Shortness of breath

- Sore throat

- Weakness

Some side effects, like high blood pressure, can occur with any NRT, because they are due to the action of the nicotine. Others—coughing, mouth and throat irritation, a stuffy or runny nose, and an upset stomach—are very common when you begin using the inhaler. However, if use is continued, the inhaler-specific symptoms usually go away. If these symptoms persist, or if you experience problems such as shortness of breath, contact your physician to determine if it is safe for you to continue using this NRT. Contact your physician *immediately* if you have any of the following problems, which may be signs of nicotine overdose.

- Abnormal heartbeat or rhythm

- Cold sweats

- Difficulty breathing

- Seizures

- Severe abdominal pain

- Tremors

The lists of potential side effects presented above are not meant to scare you, but to make you aware of the possible consequences of nicotine use or overdose so that you will be alert to problems. Similarly, it's important to understand fully that *you should not smoke when using the nicotine inhaler or any other NRT*. This can cause a serious nicotine overdose, which can result in death.

In addition to being aware of the potential side effects of the inhaler, it makes sense to understand its few drawbacks. First, as you already know, the inhaler is not as readily available as, say, nicotine gum, because you need a prescription. Second, it is not totally inconspicuous like the patch, nor can it masquerade as candy or cough drops like nicotine gum and

---

The Pros and Cons of the Nicotine Inhaler

The Pros

❏ It lessens withdrawal symptoms and cravings by supplying nicotine.

❏ Because it delivers nicotine only when used, it can help mimic the highs and lows of cigarette smoking.

❏ Through a familiar hand-to-mouth ritual, it acts as a replacement for cigarettes.

❏ It may be covered by your insurance.

The Cons

❏ You need a prescription to get it.

❏ Because it's a drug, people with certain medical problems cannot use it.

❏ It must be used carefully, and can cause side effects.

❏ It's conspicuous.

❏ A lot of hard puffing is necessary to get the nicotine you need to fight cravings and withdrawal symptoms.

lozenges. This high visibility bothers some people. Finally, some people feel that you have to work too hard to get a given amount of nicotine from the inhaler. This may make it difficult for you to get the nicotine you need to ease withdrawal symptoms and fight cravings.

CONCLUSION

Available by prescription, the nicotine inhaler can help you quit smoking cold turkey by reducing or eliminating your withdrawal symptoms. Despite the inhaler's drawbacks and possible side effects, many people have already used this type of nicotine replacement therapy safely and effectively, and some smokers prefer it because it acts as a cigarette substitute. As mentioned earlier, studies show that the inhaler can actually *double* your chance of successfully quitting the smoking habit.

Just keep in mind that like any aid, the inhaler will be effective only if you pair it with motivation and willpower. No form of nicotine replacement therapy can quit smoking for you, but if you access your core values and cement your motivation before your Quit Date, the inhaler can certainly help you get through the quitting process.

Remember, too, that this inhaler is not the only quit-smoking aid available. For that reason, before settling on an aid, you may want to consider some of the other options available. Perhaps you would have more success if you used another type of NRT, such as the patch. Or perhaps you can maximize your success by using the inhaler along with another tool, such as hypnosis. The other chapters in Part Two are packed with information about additional quit-smoking aids that can help you as you move towards a smoke-free lifestyle.

#8

Zyban

Sometimes a medication designed to provide one benefit turns out to offer other benefits, as well. This was the case with Zyban—a medication also known by its generic name, bupropion. Originally the drug was packaged in 1989 under the brand name Wellbutrin and prescribed as an antidepressant. But when smokers took the drug for depression, they reported a decreased desire for cigarettes. In fact, some people actually quit smoking without having planned to do so! Studies were then performed to investigate the medication's ability to help people stop smoking, and in 1998, the quit-smoking aid Zyban was born.

Zyban works differently from the various forms of nicotine replacement therapy (NRT) discussed in Chapters 3 through 7. It is also *used* quite differently from the NRTs. This chapter explores Zyban so that you can decide if it may be right for you.

WHAT IS IT?

Zyban is a prescription anti-smoking medication in pill form. The active ingredient in Zyban is bupropion, which was originally marketed as an antidepressant. However, this drug is chemically unrelated to other antidepressants, such as selective serotonin reuptake inhibitors and tricyclics. Each Zyban pill contains 150 milligrams of bupropion in a sustained-release formula.

This medication is intended to be used on a regular basis to minimize withdrawal symptoms and cravings.

HOW DOES IT WORK?

As you learned earlier in the book, the nicotine in cigarettes provides feelings of enjoyment by increasing brain levels of the chemical dopamine—a substance associated with the pleasure system of the brain. As nicotine creates a feeling of pleasure time and time again, it also creates an addiction that causes your brain to punish you when smoking stops. When the supply of tobacco is severed, you experience symptoms such as irritability, frustration, anxiety, restlessness, and insomnia. Many people find these symptoms so distressing that they start smoking cigarettes again despite their desire to quit.

Zyban helps you quit smoking by reducing both the symptoms of nicotine withdrawal and the craving for tobacco. It is not understood how Zyban has these effects, but it is believed that the drug affects levels of the brain's neurotransmitters—chemical messengers such as dopamine. It does *not* affect nicotine levels in the body, and contains no nicotine itself. As an added benefit, Zyban has been found to limit the weight gain that often follows smoking cessation.

Be aware that it takes about a week before Zyban begins working, and that you may need up to four weeks of treatment before you feel the full effects of the drug.

HOW DO YOU USE IT?

As you know, Zyban is a prescription medication, so you must discuss this quitting tool with your doctor and—if Zyban appears to be a safe option for you—obtain a prescription. Depending on your health insurance, this medication may or may not be covered.

Unlike therapy with NRTs such as nicotine gum, Zyban therapy begins *before* you give up cigarettes. You usually start taking one 150-milligram pill a day for the first three days while you are still smoking. Following this, you take two 150-milligram pills a day, for a total of 300 milligrams, being sure to take the two pills at least eight hours apart. Zyban therapy should continue for seven to twelve weeks, depending on the effect of the therapy. Generally, it is believed that if the patient has not at least reduced the number of cigarettes smoked by the seventh week of Zyban use, the medication should be discontinued.

Before you begin treatment with Zyban, you should choose a Quit Date—a date on which you will stop smoking. Smoking should stop within the first two weeks of Zyban treatment. As mentioned earlier, it takes about a week of treatment before the effects of Zyban are felt. By using the medication for several days before you quit smoking, you will make it easier to give up your cigarettes.

Be aware that Zyban is a powerful drug that can cause seizures in some people, although this is a rare side effect. Therefore, you must take Zyban with care:

● Swallow each Zyban pill whole. The pill is made so that the medicine is released slowly in the body. If you break or crush the pill, too much medicine can be released at once, increasing the risk of seizures.

● Take each pill with a full glass of water.

● Take the pills at the same times each day, and be sure to take them at least eight hours apart unless otherwise directed by your physician. This will help decrease the risk of seizures.

● If you miss a dose of Zyban, skip the missed dose and resume your regular dosing schedule at the appropriate time. Do not take two doses at once.

● Do not take more Zyban than directed by your doctor. The higher the dosage, the higher the risk of seizures.

● Do not drink alcohol while you are taking this medication, as alcohol can increase the risk of seizures.

Although Zyban can help you stop smoking and remain smoking-free, it's important to understand that this medication alone will not enable you to give up cigarettes. When you reach your Quit Date, you are most likely to enjoy success if you anticipate possible problems and have some solutions on hand. The following tips should help you succeed, and further guide you in using Zyban safely.

❏ As discussed in Part One (see page 28), you will more effectively use *any* method of quitting if before beginning, you identify your core values. For instance, your core value may be maintaining good health so that you can continue to participate in your favorite sports throughout your life. If you remember this core value and keep it foremost in your mind, it will be all the easier for you to keep away from cigarettes.

❏ If possible, get help from a stop-smoking program that includes either individual or group counseling. These programs—which provide encouragement and guide you in avoiding common mistakes—can double your chance of success. (See page 34 for more information.)

❏ Tell friends and family members that you have quit, and reach out to them for help when you need it. Some smokers use cigarettes as their support. If this is true of you, now is the time to make a change. I think you'll find that humans make a far better support group than a pack of cigarettes.

❏ If you miss having a cigarette in your mouth, try toothpicks, cinnamon sticks, lollipops or other hard candy, sugar-free gum, or carrot or celery sticks.

❏ If you miss holding a cigarette in your hand, replace it with a pencil, a paper clip, a marble, or a bottle of water.

❏ Keep your hands (and your mind) busy. Do crossword puzzles or needlework; try sketching or painting; clean closets; do woodworking or gardening.

❏ Try to avoid your usual triggers. If you always light up when taking a coffee break with your coworkers, skip your usual break routine and, instead, take a walk or catch up on your reading. If you enjoy a cigarette at the dinner table after your meal, get up from the table as soon as you finish eating. Cigarette smoking is a habit as well as an addiction, and habits can be broken.

❏ When a craving hits—and they *can* hit, even while you're taking Zyban—close your eyes and count slowly down from ten to zero, breathing deeply with each count. If that doesn't work, call a friend or take a walk, even if it's just to the end of your driveway. The trick is to find some diversion until the craving passes. And it will.

❏ If you're concerned about gaining weight as the result of quitting, Zyban may help, as it can reduce appetite. If not, be sure to keep healthy foods within easy reach. Those vegetable sticks will not only keep your hands busy but will also help you deal with the hunger that often results when the appetite-suppressant action of cigarettes is no longer at work. Also drink plenty of water and eat plenty of fresh fruit.

❏ Exercise. It will keep both your hands and your mind busy, providing a healthy distraction from any cravings. In fact, exercise can support your quit-smoking efforts in many ways. (To learn more, see "Exercise—A Powerful Tool Against Smoking" on page 44.)

❏ If the sight of other people smoking makes you want to reach for a cigarette, stop, and make a mental switch as discussed in Part One. (See page 36.) Instead of focusing on the great time the smokers appear to be having, think of how those cigarettes are flooding their bodies with toxins. Now picture your empty wallet, and remember what it's like to wake up with a smoker's cough. Finally, reconnect with your core values and use those values to strengthen your resolve.

❑ Resist the urge to have "just one more cigarette." Once you quit, *you quit*. And as you may already know, "one more cigarette" often increases cravings and leads to many more cigarettes.

❑ If Zyban does not sufficiently help you resist cravings or combat withdrawal symptoms, speak to your doctor about using it along with a form of nicotine replacement therapy, such as the patch or nicotine gum. Many people have found this helpful. Do not, however, combine two quitting tools without speaking to your doctor. Also remember that *you must quit smoking before using any NRT.*

❑ Keep Zyban out of the reach of children and pets.

Remember that even when using Zyban, quitting will require iron resolve. Zyban does not eliminate your emotional attachment to cigarettes, and it does not fully eliminate cravings. Don't expect quitting to be a walk in the park just because you're using Zyban. But if you're determined to quit and you want a medication to reduce withdrawal symptoms and cravings, Zyban may be the answer.

HOW WELL DOES IT WORK?

Smoking is an addiction, and the addiction is different for every person. For that reason, the withdrawal process is more difficult for some smokers than it is for others even when Zyban is in use. But evidence shows that Zyban can be effective. After a year, Zyban seems to be about twice as effective as quitting cold turkey without any aids. In other words, Zyban is about as effective as nicotine replacement therapy. Taking both Zyban and an NRT under the direction of a physician can further increase the chance of successfully quitting smoking.

RISKS AND DISADVANTAGES

Zyban is generally well tolerated. However, it's impossible to overemphasize the fact that it is a powerful prescription drug, and that it must be used exactly as your doctor recommends.

Before you start treatment, your doctor should take a complete medical history to make sure that Zyban is a safe option for you. Be sure to tell your doctor if you are pregnant, planning to become pregnant, or nursing, or if you have one of the following conditions:

- Allergies

- Anorexia nervosa, bulimia, or another eating disorder

- Cardiovascular disease, including congestive heart failure and recent heart attack

- Diabetes

- Epilepsy or another seizure disorder

- High blood pressure

- Kidney problems

- Liver problems, such as cirrhosis

- Mental or mood disorders such as depression or bipolar disorder (manic depression)

One or more of the above conditions won't necessarily rule out the use of Zyban. In the case of heart, liver, or kidney disease, for instance, your doctor may simply recommend a lower dose of the drug, or may monitor your condition throughout your Zyban therapy. In other cases, though, your physician may recommend a product that's a better match for your individual risk profile.

When discussing the possible use of Zyban with your doctor, be sure to mention all the medications you're currently taking, including prescription drugs and over-the-counter medications, as Zyban can interact with many medications. Especially tell your doctor if you are using one of the following:

- Amantadine

- Antiarrhythmics (Propafenone and others)

- Antidepressants, including monoamine oxidase inhibitors (Marplan, Nardil, Parnate, and others), tricyclics (Elavil, Tofranil, and others), and selective serotonin reuptake inhibitors (Paxil, Prozac, Zoloft, and others).

- Antipsychotics (Haldol, Thorazine, and others)

- Beta-blockers (Inderal and others)

- Bupropion (Wellbutrin)

- Carbamazepine (Epitol, Tegretol)

- Corticosteroids (Prednisone and others)

- HIV protease inhibitors

- Insulin

- Levodopa

- Oral hypoglycemics (glipizide and others)

- Phenobarbital

- Phenothiazines (Mellaril and others)

- Phenytoin

- Sympathomimetics (pseudoephedrine and others)

- Theophylline

- Tiagabine

Again, use of any of the above substances doesn't necessarily rule out the use of Zyban. But in some cases, your doctor may suggest a different quitting technique, as drug interactions can increase the risk of Zyban's side effects, can increase the side effects of the other drug, or can decrease Zyban's effectiveness.

Several substances can specifically increase the risk of seizures. These include:

- Alcohol

- Decongestants (pseudoephedrine)

- Diet pills

Do not take any of the above medications without first checking with your doctor. If you already drink alcohol or use sedatives, do not suddenly stop them without first talking to your physician. Sudden cessation may also increase seizure risk.

Like all drugs, Zyban can cause side effects. The most common side effects include the following:

- Anxiety or agitation
- Constipation
- Diarrhea
- Dizziness
- Drowsiness
- Dry mouth
- Headache
- Insomnia
- Loss of appetite
- Nausea
- Nervousness
- Shakiness
- Stomach pain
- Stuffy nose
- Weight loss

If you have trouble sleeping—a very common side effect of Zyban treatment—you may be taking a dose too close to bedtime. Talk to your doctor about changing your dosing schedule, being sure to keep the doses at least eight hours apart. Some of the problems listed above may disappear after your body adjusts to the drug. If any of these side effects persists or becomes bothersome, though, check with your doctor. Contact your physician *immediately* if you experience any of the following serious side effects:

- Blurred vision
- Breathing difficulty
- Chest pain
- Confusion
- Fast or irregular heartbeat
- Fever or chills
- Hallucinations

- Hearing problems
- Itching
- Joint or muscle pain
- Lightheadedness
- Panic attacks
- Rash
- Seizures
- Suicidal thoughts
- Tremors

The Pros and Cons of Zyban

The Pros

❏ It begins working before you give up cigarettes, priming you to stop smoking.

❏ After quitting, it lessens withdrawal symptoms and cravings.

❏ It's easy to use.

❏ It can be used inconspicuously.

❏ It can limit the weight gain associated with smoking cessation.

❏ It may be covered by your insurance.

The Cons

❏ You need a prescription to get it.

❏ Because it's a drug, people with certain medical problems cannot use it.

❏ It must be used carefully, and can cause side effects.

❏ It provides no cigarette substitute—nothing to hold in your hand or place in your mouth.

❏ It can take a week to begin working, and several weeks before the full effects are felt.

The lists of potential side effects and warning signs presented on earlier pages are not meant to scare you, but to make you aware of the possible consequences of Zyban use so that you will be alert to problems. The fact is that many people experience no side effects, or only minor or transitory problems.

In addition to being aware of the potential side effects of Zyban, it makes sense to understand its drawbacks. First, as you already know, Zyban is not as readily available as some techniques because you need a prescription to buy it. Second, Zyban takes about a week before it starts working, and sometimes several weeks before it reaches peak strength. You will have to be patient. The final drawback is that Zyban doesn't give you anything to do with your hands and mouth. If you miss holding a cigarette in your hand or putting one in your mouth, another aid, such as the nicotine inhaler, may be a better choice.

CONCLUSION

Available by prescription, Zyban can help you stop smoking cigarettes by reducing cravings and lessening your withdrawal symptoms. Despite the drug's drawbacks and possible side effects, many people have used it safely and effectively. As mentioned earlier, studies have shown that Zyban can actually *double* your chance of successfully quitting the smoking habit.

Just keep in mind that like any aid, Zyban will be effective only if you pair it with motivation and willpower. No medication can quit for you, but if you access your core values and cement your motivation, Zyban can certainly help you get through the quitting process.

Remember, too, that Zyban is not the only aid available to help you stop smoking. Perhaps you would do better with another tool entirely, or perhaps you would find it most effective to use Zyban with an NRT—a combination that many physicians advocate. The other chapters in Part Two are packed with information about additional quitting aids that can help you as you move towards a smoke-free lifestyle.

#9

Chantix

For decades, smokers in Eastern Europe have used cytisine—a medication derived from a plant called *Cytisus laburnum*—to end their dependence on tobacco. Although a number of studies documented the effectiveness of cytisine, the studies weren't published in English, so for many years, scientists in English-speaking countries were unaware of this tool in the war against smoking.

Then in 2006, the drug Chantix was introduced in the United States as a new quitting aid for smokers—the first one to be released in several years. And interestingly, the active ingredient in Chantix had been derived from the same plant that gave Europeans their drug, cytisine.

Like Zyban, discussed in Chapter 8, Chantix works differently from nicotine replacement therapy (NRT), and is also used differently from the NRTs. More important, studies show that this drug may be more effective than some popular quitting aids. Could Chantix work for you? This chapter will help you decide.

WHAT IS IT?

Chantix is a prescription anti-smoking medication in pill form. The active ingredient in Chantix is varenicline, which is also the generic name of this drug. Chantix is available in starter packs, which include pills in both 0.5-milligram and 1-milligram strengths; and in maintenance packs, which include only 1-milligram pills.

This medication is intended for use on a regular basis to make smoking less enjoyable and to minimize withdrawal symptoms and cravings.

HOW DOES IT WORK?

As you learned earlier in the book, the nicotine in cigarettes provides feelings of enjoyment by increasing brain levels of the chemical dopamine—a substance associated with the pleasure system of the brain. As nicotine creates a feeling of pleasure time and time again, it also creates an addiction that causes your brain to punish you when smoking stops. When the supply of tobacco is severed, you experience symptoms such as irritability, frustration, anxiety, restlessness, and insomnia. Many people find these symptoms so distressing that they start smoking cigarettes again despite their desire to quit.

Chantix acts on a neurological level to help you quit smoking in two ways. First, it actually blocks some of the effects of nicotine, making the smoking experience less pleasurable. Initially, this makes it easier to give up cigarettes; and later, if you slip and resume smoking, it makes it far easier to stop at a few puffs. Second, Chantix mimics the action of nicotine to increase levels of dopamine, thus easing withdrawal symptoms. Chantix does not affect nicotine levels in the body, contains no nicotine itself, and is not an antidepressant like Zyban. But like Zyban, Chantix does take some time to begin working.

HOW DO YOU USE IT?

Because Chantix is a prescription medication, you must discuss this quitting tool with your doctor and—if Chantix appears to be a safe option for you—obtain a prescription. Depending on your health insurance, this medication may or may not be covered.

It is recommended that before you start using Chantix, you pick a Quit Date—a date on which you will stop smoking. Seven days before your Quit Date, you usually start taking one 0.5-milligram tablet of Chantix each day. On day four, you take two 0.5-milligram tablets each day—one in the morning and one in the evening. Starting on day seven, you begin taking two 1-milligram tablets each day—one in the morning and one in the evening. This gradual increase in dosage is intended to reduce the chance of side effects in general, and specifically minimize the most common side effect of nausea. To further decrease your chance of experiencing nausea and other problems, be sure to do the following:

- Take each pill with a full glass of water.
- Take each pill after eating.

• If you miss a dose, take it as soon as you remember. If it is close to the time for your next dose, wait, and take your regular dose at the proper time. Do not take two doses together.

• Do not take more Chantix than directed by your doctor. The higher the dosage, the higher the incidence of side effects.

Although the dosing schedule discussed earlier is recommended by the manufacturer and is effective for many people, it may not be right for everyone. If you find yourself having side effects, check with your doctor. He or she may want to reduce your dose.

Ideally, you will stop smoking on the seventh day of treatment, after Chantix has had some time to build up in your body. It's important to at least try to stop smoking on your Quit Date. If you slip, try again. In some cases, it takes several weeks for Chantix to reach full strength. Most people keep taking Chantix for twelve weeks. But if you successfully quit smoking during that first course of treatment, your doctor may prescribe a second twelve-week course of treatment to better ensure your long-term success.

Although Chantix can help you stop smoking and remain smoking-free, it's important to understand that this medication alone will not enable you to give up cigarettes. When you reach your Quit Date, you are most likely to enjoy success if you anticipate possible problems and have some solutions on hand. The following tips should help you succeed, and also guide you in using Chantix safely:

❑ As discussed in Part One (see page 28), you will more effectively use *any* method of quitting if before beginning, you identify your core values. For instance, your core value may be maintaining good health so that you can continue to participate in your favorite sports throughout your life. If you remember this core value and keep it foremost in your mind, it will be all the easier for you to keep away from cigarettes.

❑ If possible, get help from a stop-smoking program that includes either individual or group counseling. These programs—which provide encouragement and guide you in avoiding common mistakes—can double your chance of success. (See page 34 for more information.)

❑ Tell friends and family members that you have quit, and reach out to them for help when you need it. Some smokers use cigarettes as their support. If this is true of you, now is the time to make a change. I think you'll find that humans make a far better support group than a pack of cigarettes.

❑ If you miss having a cigarette in your mouth, try toothpicks, cinnamon sticks, lollipops or other hard candy, sugar-free gum, or carrot or celery sticks.

❑ If you miss holding a cigarette in your hand, replace it with a pencil, a paper clip, a marble, or a bottle of water.

❑ Keep your hands (and your mind) busy. Do crossword puzzles or needlework; try sketching or painting; clean closets; do woodworking or gardening.

❑ Try to avoid your usual triggers. If you always light up when taking a coffee break with your coworkers, skip your usual break routine and, instead, take a walk or catch up on your reading. If you enjoy a cigarette at the dinner table after your meal, get up from the table as soon as you finish eating. Smoking is a habit as well as an addiction, and habits can be broken.

❑ When a craving hits—and they *can* hit, even while you're taking Chantix—close your eyes and count slowly down from ten to zero, breathing deeply with each count. If that doesn't work, call a friend or take a walk, even if it's just to the end of your driveway. The trick is to find some diversion until the craving passes. And it will.

❑ If you're concerned about gaining weight as the result of quitting, Chantix may or may not help. While some people report increased appetite when using Chantix, others do not. If you find yourself eating more after you quit smoking, be sure to keep healthy foods within easy reach. Those vegetable sticks will not only keep your hands busy but will also help you deal with the hunger that often results when the appetite-suppressant action of cigarettes is no longer at work. Also drink plenty of water and eat plenty of fresh fruit.

❑ Exercise. It will keep both your hands and your mind busy, providing a healthy distraction from any cravings. In fact, exercise can support your quit-smoking efforts in many ways. (To learn more, see "Exercise—A Powerful Tool Against Smoking" on page 44.)

❑ If the sight of other people smoking makes you want to reach for a cigarette, stop, and make a mental switch as discussed in Part One. (See page 36.) Instead of focusing on the great time the smokers appear to be having, think of how those cigarettes are flooding their bodies with toxins. Now picture your empty wallet, and remember what it's like to wake up with a smoker's cough. Finally, reconnect with your core values and use those values to strengthen your resolve.

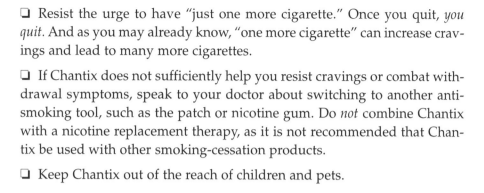

❏ Resist the urge to have "just one more cigarette." Once you quit, *you quit*. And as you may already know, "one more cigarette" can increase cravings and lead to many more cigarettes.

❏ If Chantix does not sufficiently help you resist cravings or combat withdrawal symptoms, speak to your doctor about switching to another anti-smoking tool, such as the patch or nicotine gum. Do *not* combine Chantix with a nicotine replacement therapy, as it is not recommended that Chantix be used with other smoking-cessation products.

❏ Keep Chantix out of the reach of children and pets.

Keep in mind that even when using Chantix, quitting will require iron resolve. Chantix does not eliminate your emotional attachment to cigarettes, and it does not fully eliminate cravings. Don't expect quitting to be a walk in the park just because you're using Chantix. But if you're determined to stop smoking and you want a medication that reduces withdrawal symptoms and cravings, Chantix may be the answer.

HOW WELL DOES IT WORK?

Smoking is an addiction, and the addiction is different for every person. For that reason, the withdrawal process is more difficult for some than it is for others even when Chantix is in use. But evidence shows that Chantix can be effective. According to studies, Chantix may be nearly *three times* as effective as quitting cold turkey without any aids. Moreover, some studies have shown Chantix to be more effective than Zyban.

While the above information is promising, it's important to be aware that results have been mixed. One study indicated that Chantix works better than Zyban for only the first twenty-four weeks after quitting; another, that Chantix works better for more than a year. No studies have yet compared the effectiveness of Chantix either with that of nicotine replacement therapy, or with that of Zyban and an NRT combined.

RISKS AND DISADVANTAGES

As you know, many people have experienced quitting success with the help of Chantix. But it's impossible to overemphasize the fact that it is a powerful prescription drug, and that it must be used exactly as your doctor recommends.

The Pros and Cons of Chantix

The Pros

❏ Before quitting, it reduces the enjoyment of cigarettes, helping you to stop smoking.

❏ After quitting, it lessens withdrawal symptoms and cravings, and—if you slip—it makes smoking less pleasurable.

❏ It's easy to use.

❏ It can be used inconspicuously.

❏ It may be covered by your insurance.

The Cons

❏ You need a prescription to get it.

❏ Because it's a drug, it must be used carefully and can cause side effects, especially nausea.

❏ It provides no cigarette substitute—nothing to hold in your hand or place in your mouth.

❏ It can take a week or more to begin working, and several weeks before the full effects are felt.

Before you start treatment, your doctor should take a complete medical history and perform a physical examination to make sure that Chantix is a safe option for you. Be sure to tell your doctor if you are pregnant, planning to become pregnant, or nursing; or if you have kidney problems or are currently on kidney dialysis. It is not known if Chantix can harm an unborn baby if used during pregnancy, or if it passes into breast milk, but it is suggested that the drug be avoided in these cases. If you have a kidney problem, your doctor may recommend a lower dose of Chantix, or may suggest that you avoid using this drug. Some physicians test kidney function on a regular basis throughout treatment to make sure that the medication is causing no harmful effects.

When discussing the possible use of Chantix with your doctor, be sure to mention all the medications you're currently taking, including prescription drugs and over-the-counter-medications. Especially tell your doctor if you are using one of the following:

- Asthma medication

- Blood thinners

- Insulin

According to clinical experience to date, Chantix has no significant drug interactions, which means that when you add Chantix to any medication you're taking, no adverse reactions should take place. However, as you stop smoking, there may be a change in how certain drugs—especially those listed above—work for you. For that reason, dosage adjustments may have to be made.

Like all drugs, Chantix can cause side effects. The most common side effects include the following:

- Abdominal pain

- Change in taste perception

- Constipation

- Excess gas (flatulence)

- Fatigue or weakness

- Headache

- Insomnia or abnormal dreams

- Increased appetite

- Nausea

- Vomiting

As you learned earlier, nausea is the most common side effect among Chantix users. In various studies, 30 to 40 percent of users reported this symptom, with most of them experiencing mild or moderate nausea. For some people, the nausea abated after their body adjusted to the medication, but some users experienced persistent nausea throughout treatment. If this or any other side effect becomes bothersome, or if you experience unusual symptoms, be sure to check with your doctor. Contact your physician *immediately* if you experience any of the following signs of an allergic reaction:

- Breathing difficulty

- Hives

- Swelling of face, lips, tongue, or throat

The lists of potential side effects and warning signs presented above are not meant to scare you, but to make you aware of the possible consequences of Chantix use so that you will be alert to problems. The fact is that many people experience no side effects, or have only minor or transitory problems that don't prevent them from continuing treatment

In addition to being aware of the potential side effects of Chantix, it makes sense to understand its drawbacks. First, as you know, Chantix is not as readily available as some anti-smoking techniques because you need a prescription to buy it. Second, Chantix takes a week or more to reach full strength and effectiveness. You will have to be patient. The final drawback is that Chantix doesn't give you anything to do with your hands and mouth. If you miss holding a cigarette in your hand or putting one in your mouth, another aid, such as the nicotine inhaler, may be a better choice.

CONCLUSION

Available by prescription, Chantix can help you quit smoking by lessening the pleasure felt when smoking cigarettes, and by reducing cravings and withdrawal symptoms. Despite the drug's drawbacks and possible side effects, many people have used it safely and effectively. As mentioned earlier, studies have shown that Chantix may nearly *triple* your chance of successfully quitting the smoking habit, and may be more effective than the anti-smoking medication Zyban.

Just keep in mind that like any aid, Chantix will be effective only if you pair it with motivation and willpower. No medication can quit for you, but if you access your core values and cement your motivation, Chantix can certainly help you get through the quitting process.

Remember, too, that Chantix is not the only aid available to help you stop smoking. If you read earlier chapters, you've already learned about nicotine replacement therapy and Zyban. In the next chapter, you'll learn about hypnosis—an anti-smoking tool that can be used alone, or paired with medication to help you successfully move towards a smoke-free lifestyle.

#10

Hypnosis

A century ago, hypnosis was viewed as a mental state imposed on an individual by a "Svengali," who sought to exercise complete control over his victim. A half century ago, the average person regarded hypnosis as a type of magic act in which the hypnotist would cause someone to cluck like a chicken, or otherwise act in a ridiculous manner, as a means of entertainment. Now, hypnosis—or, more precisely, *hypnotherapy*—is used to help people deal with a range of health and behavioral problems, including the addiction to tobacco. Hypnotists abound, promising to help you throw away your cigarettes forever.

Just how does hypnosis work? And, perhaps more important, *does* it work as an effective anti-smoking tool? That is the subject of this chapter.

WHAT IS IT?

So far, science has been unable to explain exactly what hypnosis is. Most often, it is described as a mental state characterized by extreme suggestibility, relaxation, and heightened imagination. Although the word *hypnosis* comes from the Greek word *hypnos*, meaning sleep, hypnosis is not like sleep, because you are alert throughout the process. Often, it is compared to daydreaming in that you are fully conscious, but have tuned out most of the stimuli around you. Instead of being distracted by your surroundings or by everyday concerns and activities, you are intensely focused on the subject at hand—the subject to which the hypnotist draws your attention.

How can hypnosis help you kick the habit? Practitioners of hypnotism have found that when you are in a hypnotic state, the critical side of your brain—the conscious part—has, in effect, been shut off. Your subconscious is therefore able to accept posthypnotic suggestions as fact. And when the hypnotic state ends and you are in a waking state, the suggestions remain in your subconscious, helping to mold both your thinking and your behavior. So through hypnosis, information that is detrimental to your well-being, such as the belief that smoking feels great, can be replaced with information that can lead to a healthy, smoke-free life. When hypnosis is used in this way, to treat a health condition, it is referred to as *hypnotherapy.*

HOW DOES IT WORK?

Most people find the idea of hypnosis a little foreign, or even frightening, simply because they don't know what happens during a hypnotherapy session. Fortunately, this is not a mystery.

A good hypnotherapist will begin by learning about you. Why do you want to give up smoking? What negative things in your life—coughing, high expenses, the inability to participate in sports as you'd like—are associated with smoking cigarettes? What positive things—greater health, more money for travel, being able to play a great game of tennis—do you associate with quitting? This information can help the hypnotist create posthypnotic suggestions and visualizations that are meaningful to you.

Can You Be Hypnotized?

Many people are intrigued by the idea of hypnotherapy, but never try it simply because they believe that they can't be hypnotized. They may have heard that only some people can be put in a trance state, or they may assume that they have too much willpower to "go under."

The fact is that unless you don't want to be hypnotized, you can be. However, different people can be hypnotized to different degrees. A small percentage of people—about one in five—can be so deeply hypnotized that they see, hear, and feel imaginary things as if they were real. Other people have less vivid, less realistic experiences during hypnosis. But even the person who goes into a very deep trance state understands that the illusions are just illusions.

Can *you* be hypnotized? Yes, if you want to be. Can hypnosis help you quit smoking? Well, hypnosis can't make you do anything you don't want to do. But if you have a strong desire to give up cigarettes, but just can't get through the quitting process, you may find that hypnosis is the tool you've been looking for.

Contrary to what you may believe, most people *can* be hypnotized. (For more about this, see "Can You Be Hypnotized?" on page 132.) Hypnotists have a number of ways to guide patients into a trance state. Most people have seen the eye fixation method in movies, where the hypnotist waves a shiny pocket watch in front of his subject. While this is a valid technique, it is rarely used because it works on only a small portion of the population. Today, most hypnotists use progressive relaxation and imagery to bring about a trance state. If your hypnotist employs this method, he or she will speak to you in a slow, soothing voice to gradually relax you, focus your attention, and bring you into full hypnosis.

When you are under hypnosis, and your conscious mind is no longer in charge, the hypnotist will be able to directly access your subconscious mind, which is just below the level of consciousness. He or she can then address your habit of smoking and help reverse your behavior by reprogramming your subconscious. This, too, can be done in various ways. For instance, the hypnotist might suggest that every time you feel like smoking a cigarette, you drink a glass of water instead. This, in effect, would replace an old habit with a new healthier habit—perhaps a habit that you told him you'd like to acquire. He or she may further suggest that every time you drink that water, you feel great—strong, fit, and happy.

Posthypnotic suggestions can also be used to change your opinion of cigarettes. Perhaps you will be told that every time you think of smoking a cigarette, you will remember that you are *not* a smoker, and that cigarettes are vile to you—foul tasting, bad smelling, and generally revolting. The hypnotist may even tell you that smoking causes nausea so that you feel ill every time you think of cigarettes.

Posthypnotic suggestions can also be used to build up your willpower. Your hypnotist may suggest that you don't need cigarettes and that you don't want them. You are tougher than tobacco.

When the session is nearing its end, the hypnotist usually uses a simple word or suggestion to bring you out of the hypnotic state. If you are like most people, you will be able to remember both what you said and what the hypnotist said to you during the session.

HOW DO YOU USE IT?

If you are interested in using hypnosis to kick your smoking habit, your first task is to find a reputable hypnotist who is experienced in helping people stop smoking. You may already be aware that some quit-smoking hypnosis is performed on groups, but studies show that the greatest success is experienced by smokers who work with a good practitioner on a one-to-one basis. (See "Choosing a Qualified Hypnotist" on page 135.) This arrangement allows the hypnotist to design a hypnotherapy session specifically for you.

Recognize that the date of your hypnosis session is also your Quit Date, and set the stage for success. Before going to your session, throw out your cigarettes, matches, and lighters, and commit yourself to quitting cold turkey. It doesn't make much sense to drive away from your hypnotist's office in a car stocked with cigarettes and matches.

Finally, don't make the mistake of thinking that hypnosis will do the quitting for you. Yes, hypnotherapy can be a wonderful anti-smoking tool, but you still have to be strongly motivated and ready to work if you want to beat your dependency on cigarettes. These tips should help:

❑ As discussed in Part One (see page 28), you will more effectively use *any* method of quitting if before beginning, you identify your core values. For instance, your core value may be maintaining good health so that you can be an active part of your children's lives, and see them grow up and have children of their own. If you remember this core value and keep it foremost in your mind, it will be all the easier for you to walk past the convenience store without running in for a pack of cigarettes. In fact, you will *have* to walk past it in order to remain true to yourself.

❑ If possible, get help from a stop-smoking program that includes either individual or group counseling. These programs—which provide encouragement and guide you in avoiding common mistakes—can double your chance of success. (See page 34 for more information.)

❑ Tell friends and family members that you have quit, and reach out to them for help when you need it. Some smokers use cigarettes as their support. If this is true of you, now is the time to make a change. I think you'll find that humans make a far better support group than a pack of cigarettes.

❑ If you miss having a cigarette in your mouth, try toothpicks, cinnamon sticks, lollipops or other hard candy, sugar-free gum, or carrot or celery sticks.

❑ If you miss holding a cigarette in your hand, replace it with a pencil, a paper clip, a marble, or a bottle of water.

❑ Keep your hands (and your mind) busy. Do crossword puzzles or needlework; try sketching or painting; clean closets; do woodworking or gardening.

Choosing a Qualified Hypnotist

Hypnosis can be a powerful tool in the war against smoking. But it can be effective only if your hypnotist is a capable professional.

To find a qualified hypnotist, start by asking friends and family members if they have used a local hypnotist to successfully quit smoking or fight another bad habit, such as overeating. If the people you know can't provide any leads, speak to your primary physician to see if he or she can recommend a hypnotist. Although many doctors know little about hypnosis, your doctor's experience in working with other smokers may have made him aware of good professionals in the area.

If no one offers a personal recommendation, and you have to find a hypnotist on your own, start by contacting professional organizations such as the American Society of Clinical Hypnosis and the National Guild of Hypnotists. They should be able to refer you to certified practitioners in your area. (See page 145 of the Resources section for contact information.) Of course, you can also search the Internet or turn to the Yellow Pages.

Once you have located a name or two, you'll want to call the hypnotist's office and ask some questions. You should be able to gauge if the hypnotist is interested in your concerns, and if he or she is experienced in working with smokers. Be sure to ask if you will receive either a tape of your session or a pre-made tape that can be used for reinforcement at home. Whether the tape is generic or geared especially for you, it can be a great means of supporting the office hypnotherapy session and helping you keep on track. Also ask if the hypnotist will provide free follow-up sessions if you start slipping in the future. Finally, request the names of satisfied patients who have worked with that hypnotist. An experienced, competent professional should have a long list of clients who will gladly speak to you about their experiences.

If you're pleased with the answers you receive, you can feel good about making an appointment. Try to approach your session with an open mind and the desire to work with the hypnotist, as this will yield the best results. If you're like most people, you will come out of your session feeling relaxed, positive, and full of motivation for the task ahead.

❏ Try to avoid your usual triggers. If you always light up when taking a coffee break with your coworkers, skip your usual break routine and, instead, take a walk or catch up on your reading. If you enjoy a cigarette at the dinner table after your meal, get up from the table as soon as you finish eating. Cigarette smoking is a habit as well as an addiction, and habits can be broken.

❑ When a craving hits—and it can, even if you've gone through hypnosis—close your eyes and count slowly down from ten to zero, breathing deeply with each count. It that doesn't work, call a friend or take a walk—even if it's just to the end of your driveway. The trick is to find some diversion until the craving passes. And it will.

❑ If you're concerned about gaining weight as the result of quitting, keep healthy foods within easy reach. Those vegetable sticks will not only keep your hands busy but will also help you deal with the hunger that often results when the appetite-suppressant action of cigarettes is no longer at work. Also drink plenty of water and eat plenty of fresh fruit.

❑ Exercise. It will not only fight weight gain, but will also help calm your nerves. And it will keep both your hands and your mind busy, providing a healthy distraction from any cravings. In fact, exercise can support your quitting efforts in many ways. (To learn more, see "Exercise—A Powerful Tool Against Smoking" on page 44.)

❑ If the sight of other people smoking makes you want to reach for a cigarette, stop, and make a mental switch as discussed in Part One. (See page 36.) Instead of focusing on the great time the smokers appear to be having, think of how those cigarettes are flooding their bodies with toxins. Now picture your empty wallet, and remember what it's like to wake up with a smoker's cough. Finally, reconnect with your core values and use those values to strengthen your resolve.

❑ Don't be concerned if you find yourself coughing a great deal during the first few days of withdrawal, or even for a couple of weeks. This is actually a good sign, as your body is ridding itself of the tars and toxins that have accumulated through years of smoking. The cough won't last long, but while it's there, keep your throat as moist and comfortable as possible by drinking plenty of fluids and using throat lozenges.

❑ Resist the urge to have "just one more cigarette." Once you quit smoking, *you quit.* If you give yourself the option of having another cigarette, you will keep sliding. And every time you give in, you will have to start at the beginning again. Don't do that to yourself. Once you've made the commitment to quit, keep your commitment.

❑ To optimize your success, consider pairing hypnosis with another anti-smoking weapon, such as the nicotine patch or Zyban. Since hypnosis is not a drug, it can be safely combined with any of the NRTs or medications designed to lessen withdrawal symptoms and cravings. Studies have shown that hypnosis works best when it's combined with another quitting method.

Finally, if your hypnotist gives you a tape or CD to use at home, *use it.* Quitting is tough, and even with a good tool like hypnosis, you need all the help you can get. Take advantage of any and all aids that your hypnotist provides, and be willing to do a little work. If you feel yourself slipping, give him or her a call and ask for a follow-up session. The results will be well worth the effort.

HOW WELL DOES IT WORK?

No studies have conclusively determined the effectiveness of hypnosis as a stop-smoking tool. One group of researchers reviewed five dozen studies on the effectiveness of hypnosis for smokers who wished to quit. The researchers encountered various problems during their analysis, including the fact that there is no standard way to perform hypnosis. For instance, some studies involved single-session hypnotherapy, while others involved multiple-session hypnotherapy. Moreover, some groups of smokers were offered other anti-smoking interventions, such as the patch or counseling, in addition to hypnosis.

After all the studies were examined, the only conclusion that could be reached was that smokers who undergo hypnosis have greater success than those who have no form of intervention whatsoever, and that this tool works best when used in conjunction with other methods. More studies are needed to determine just how effective hypnosis is as a quitting aid. But no one can argue with the fact that some people do stop smoking—forever—using hypnosis and hypnosis alone.

RISKS AND DISADVANTAGES

Hypnotherapy is considered safe for everyone. Although it may not always have the effect you desire, it involves no risks. And contrary to what many people believe, it cannot make you do something you don't want to do or something that would go against your personal ethics. Of course, the best way to guard against undesired effects of *any* type is to work with a professionally trained hypnosis specialist.

The Pros and Cons of Hypnosis

The Pros

❏ It can help you strengthen your motivation and build new, healthier habits.

❏ It's drug-free, and can be used regardless of any medical problems you have and any medications you may be using.

❏ It's an inconspicuous aid.

❏ It can safely and easily be paired with both over-the-counter and prescription quitting aids, including nicotine replacement therapy, Zyban, and Chantix.

The Cons

❏ It doesn't lessen withdrawal symptoms or cravings.

❏ It provides no cigarette substitute—nothing to hold in your hand or place in your mouth.

❏ Generally, it is not covered by insurance.

The disadvantage of using hypnosis to quit smoking is that, unlike NRTs and other aids discussed earlier, it does not diminish cravings and withdrawal symptoms. It also does not act like a cigarette substitute, as the nicotine inhaler does. This may be why some people are most successful when they pair hypnosis with other smoking-cessation tools.

CONCLUSION

A good hypnotherapist can work with you closely and tailor a hypnosis session to your specific needs and goals. He or she can then use posthypnotic suggestions to replace your smoking habit with a healthful habit, help change your opinion of cigarettes, and boost your willpower, easing you through the quitting process.

Just keep in mind that like any aid, hypnotherapy will be effective only if you pair it with strong resolve. In most cases, the hypnotist cannot make quitting effortless. But if you access your core values and follow the hypnotist's directions involving tapes or other aids, hypnotherapy can help you enjoy a smoke-free life.

Conclusion

My uncle quit smoking over twenty years ago. He struggled and struggled with quitting, and he finally succeeded. When I graduated from college, he said that he'd never expected to see that day. When I graduated from medical school, we went for a long walk together, and he breathed freely and easily. Quitting saved my uncle's life. It can save yours, too.

You came to this book wanting to quit, and together, we've covered a lot of ground. You now should have a better understanding of why you started smoking in the first place, how your addiction took hold of you, and how your habit is damaging not only your own health, but also the health of those around you. Furthermore, you have hopefully taken some quiet time to consider your innermost core values. Being connected to your core values should be central to your quitting efforts. Once you have identified "being healthy" or "wanting to see your kids grow up" as a value, not smoking simply becomes a manifestation of who you are.

Armed with a fervent commitment to stop smoking, we have explored the top ten anti-smoking tools and techniques. None of these tools will do the work for you, but each can help. The key is to find the tool or combination of tools that is right for *you*, as no two smokers are exactly alike. Maybe your buddy quit using the patch, but you would do better with the nicotine inhaler because it acts as a cigarette substitute. Or perhaps you'd feel more comfortable avoiding nicotine altogether and choosing an aid such as Chantix. The boxed Pros and Cons insets found in each of the ten techniques chapters should make it easier for you to find a method or combination of methods that addresses your particular needs and preferences.

While you are the captain of your quit-smoking ship, never forget that to reach your journey's end, you need a good crew. That's why it's essential to work with your doctor in choosing and using anti-smoking tools—especially if you want to employ a combination of aids. Just because it's *possible* to mix certain smoking-cessation aids, doesn't mean that it's safe to do so in your particular situation. So check with your physician before choosing even an over-the-counter aid, and follow his or her directions throughout the quitting process.

You may think that a support team is optional, but studies have shown that it's not. Again and again, researchers have learned that smokers enjoy greatest quitting success when they have good support. Whether it's friends and family, an online program, a telephone quitline, or a face-to-face group, your team will give you the encouragement you need to keep your spirits and motivation high. Don't make the mistake of thinking that people who reach for support are weak. Actually, they're smart—and successful.

Of course, at the end of the day, no one can quit for you. You have to do it yourself. That's why it's so important to recognize that you *can* do this—you can toss your cigarettes away and never touch another pack. Humans have built pyramids in the desert, scaled Mount Everest, overcome polio, and walked on the moon. Although it may be tough, you can climb your own personal mountain and enjoy a smoke-free life.

I wish you good luck, because we can all use a little. I wish you a favorable wind at your back, so that your journey may progress smoothly. And I wish you good health, because with health, all things are possible.

Resources

A number of organizations—both government and private—make available a wide range of information and services, from tips for smoking cessation to telephone quitlines. All of these groups offer information or other types of assistance through their websites, and some also can be contacted by phone or mail. The organizations and websites listed directly below provide general information on tobacco and smoking cessation, and in some cases, also offer support. Turn to page 143 for programs dedicated to providing smoking-cessation support, and to page 145 for organizations that can refer you to qualified hypnotherapists in your area.

GENERAL INFORMATION ORGANIZATIONS AND WEBSITES

American Cancer Society
Phone: 800-ACS-2345
Website: www.cancer.org

Created to eliminate cancer as a major health problem, the ACS provides information on nicotine, nicotine withdrawal, the dangers of tobacco, and smoking-cessation methods. Visit its website and click on "Guide to Quitting Smoking."

American Heart Association
National Center
7272 Greenville Avenue
Dallas, TX 75231
Phone: 800-242-8721
Website: www.americanheart.org

With the goal of reducing disability and death from heart disease, the American Heart Association devotes a portion of its very comprehensive website to presenting information about smoking risks, as well as links to quitting tools and resources. Click first on "Healthy Lifestyle," then on "Smoking and Cardiovascular Disease."

American Lung Association

61 Broadway, 6th Floor

New York, NY 10006

Phone: 800-LUNGUSA

Website: www.lungusa.org

Dedicated to preventing lung disease, the ALA provides a wealth of information on the benefits of quitting, smoking-cessation aids, and much more. Visit the website and click first on "Quit Smoking," then on "Smoking Cessation Support."

Centers for Disease Control and Prevention

1600 Clifton Road

Atlanta, GA 30333

Phone: 800-311-3435

Website: http://www.cdc.gov/tobacco

Established to prevent and control disease, the Centers for Disease Control and Prevention uses a portion of its website to address tobacco-related issues. There, you'll find quitting tips, Surgeon General's reports, citations from recently published articles about tobacco, educational information, and links to telephone quitlines.

National Cancer Institute

Room 3036A

6116 Executive Boulevard

Bethesda, MD 20892-9322

Phone: 800-422-6237

Website: www.cancer.gov/cancertopics/factsheet/tobacco

At the forefront of cancer research, NCI makes available a vast amount of cancer-related information. Visit its website for links to a long list of fact sheets, most of which focus on different aspects of quitting the tobacco habit.

National Library of Medicine
Reference and Web Services
8600 Rockville Pike
Bethesda, MD 20894
Phone: 888-346-3656
Website: www.nlm.nih.gov

The National Library of Medicine is the world's largest medical library. Its website, created with the National Institute of Health, provides links to health information of all types. Perform a search for "Smoking Cessation," and find tips on quitting and much more.

The Surgeon General
Office of the Surgeon General
5600 Fishers Lane
Room 18-66
Rockville, MD 20857
Phone: 301-443-4000
Website: www.surgeongeneral.gov/tobacco

The Surgeon General is America's chief health educator. Visit the Surgeon General's website to find information on quitting, telephone quitlines, Surgeon General's reports, and more.

SMOKING-CESSATION PROGRAMS AND SUPPORT GROUPS

Freedom From Smoking Online
Website: www.lungusa.org

Freedom From Smoking Online is the American Lung Association's web-based smoking cessation support program. This site will also help you find a person-to-person program in your area. When you reach the ALA's website, click first on "Quit Smoking," then on "FFS Online Program."

Nicotine Anonymous
419 Main Street, PMB #370
Huntington Beach, CA 92648
Phone: 415-750-0328
Website: www.nicotine-anonymous.org

Modeled after Alcoholics Anonymous, Nicotine Anonymous provides a twelve-step support program for people who have quit cold turkey or with nicotine replacement therapies. Check the website for program information, support, literature, and referrals to local meeting schedules and locations.

North American Quitline Consortium
4142 E. Stanford Drive
Phoenix, AZ 85018
Phone: 800-784-8669
Website: www.naquitline.com

The object of the North American Quitline Consortium is to increase access to and effectiveness of smokers' quitlines. Call the consortium for referral to a quitline that can provide you with support and counseling, smoking-cessation medications at low or no cost, printed support information, web-based interactive counseling, and more.

Quit Smoking Journals
PO Box 850
Princeton Junction, NJ 08550
Website: www.quitsmokingjournals.com

This website offers community quit-smoking support through a journaling service. Once you register, you can post your own quitting journal and read the entries of others who are working towards a tobacco-free life. Tips for effective journaling are offered by the website staff.

Quit Wizard
Website: www.trytostop.org/QuitWizardV2

This site of the Massachusetts Department of Health offers tools for personalized planning, helps you track your progress, and guides you through each phase of the quitting process.

QuitNet
Website: www.quitnet.com (quitting plan)
Website: www.quitnet.com/library/programs (directory)

Operated in association with the Boston University School of Public Health, the QuitNet website offers cessation information, helps you create a quitting plan, and provides support via chat rooms. Quitnet also maintains the

National Directory of Smoking Cessation Programs—the largest database of this type in the United States.

Smokefree.gov
Website: www.smokefree.gov

Created by the National Cancer Institute, the CDC, and other health organizations, Smokefree.gov provides information and support for those who are trying to quit smoking. The website offers an online guide to quitting; telephone support; live, online assistance from the National Cancer Institute's LiveHelp service; and an extensive list of materials that can be read online, printed out, or ordered.

Smoking Cessation Forum at About.com
Website: http://quitsmoking.about.com/mpboards.htm

The About.com smoking-cessation website provides quit-smoking support through a discussion forum. Participants can enter as a guest to read posts, or can register for free to ask questions, express opinions, and give and receive advice and encouragement.

HYPNOSIS ORGANIZATIONS AND WEBSITES

American Society of Clinical Hypnosis
140 N. Bloomingdale Road
Bloomingdale, IL 60108
Phone: 630-980-4740
Website:www.asch.net

ASCH is the largest U.S. organization for health-care professionals using clinical hypnosis. Its website allows you to search for an ASCH member by location or specialty.

National Guild of Hypnotists
PO Box 308
Merrimack, NH 03054
Phone: 603-429-9438
Website: www.ngh.net

A not-for profit professional organization, the National Guild of Hypnotists provides a website service that enables you to find NGH certified hypnotists in your area.

Index